D0188557

SUDDEN UNEXPECTED DEATHS IN INFANCY

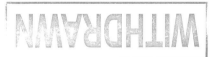
WITHDRAWN

WP 2200447 5

SUDDEN UNEXPECTED DEATHS IN INFANCY

THE CESDI SUDI STUDIES 1993–1996

Editors:
Professor Peter Fleming
Dr Chris Bacon
Dr Peter Blair
Professor PJ Berry

Contributors:
Martin Ward Platt, Iain Smith, Shireen
Chantler, Pam Mueller, Shirley Stephenson,
Eleanor Allibone, Pat McKeever, Isabelle
Moore, Chris Wright, Pam Nadin, Charlotte
Leach, John Tripp, Jean Golding and the
CESDI SUDI research team

UNIVERSITY OF WOLVERHAMPTON
LIBRARY

Acc No.
2200447

CLASS
618·
92
SUD

CONTROL
0113222998

DATE
MAY 2000

SITE
New

wL

London: The Stationery Office

© The Stationery Office 2000

All rights reserved. No part of this publication may be reproduced, stored in a retrieval system, or transmitted in any form or by any means, electronic, mechanical, photocopying, recording or otherwise without the permission of the publisher.

Applications for reproduction should be made in writing to The Stationery Office Limited, St Crispins, Duke Street, Norwich NR3 1PD.

The information contained in this publication is believed to be correct at the time of manufacture. Whilst care has been taken to ensure that the information is accurate, the publisher can accept no responsibility for any errors or omissions or for changes to the details given. Every effort has been made to trace copyright holders and to obtain permission for the use of copyright material. The publishers will gladly receive any information enabling them to rectify any errors or omissions in subsequent editions.

A CIP catalogue record for this book is available from the British Library
A Library of Congress CIP catalogue record has been applied for

First published 2000

ISBN 0 11 322299 8

Printed in the United Kingdom by Albert Gait Ltd, Grimsby, North East Lincolnshire.
J95925 C10 01/00 9385 11507

Published by The Stationery Office and available from:

The Publications Centre
(mail, telephone and fax orders only)
PO Box 276, London SW8 5DT
General enquiries/Telephone orders 0870 600 5522
Fax orders 0870 600 5533

www.tso-online.co.uk

The Stationery Office Bookshops
123 Kingsway, London WC2B 6PQ
020 7242 6393 Fax 020 7242 6412
68–69 Bull Street, Birmingham B4 6AD
0121 236 9696 Fax 0121 236 9699
33 Wine Street, Bristol BS1 2BQ
0117 926 4306 Fax 0117 929 4515
9–21 Princess Street, Manchester M60 8AS
0161 834 7201 Fax 0161 833 0634
16 Arthur Street, Belfast BT1 4GD
028 9023 8451 Fax 028 9023 5401
The Stationery Office Oriel Bookshop
18–19 High Street, Cardiff CF1 2BZ
029 2039 5548 Fax 029 2038 4347
71 Lothian Road, Edinburgh EH3 9AZ
0870 606 5566 Fax 0870 606 5588

The Stationery Office's Accredited Agents
(see Yellow Pages)

and through good booksellers

CONTENTS

THE CESDI SUDI RESEARCH TEAM (FULL LIST)

South-Western and Wessex

Professor Peter Fleming	*Professor of Infant Health and Developmental Physiology, chair of project planning and co-ordinating group*
Dr Peter Blair	*Medical Statistician*
Professor Jem Berry	*Professor of Paediatric Pathology*
Dr Isabella Moore	*Consultant Pathologist*
Professor Jean Golding	*Professor of Paediatric and Perinatal Epidemiology*
Dr John Tripp	*Senior Lecturer in Child Health*
Rosie Thompson	*CESDI Regional Coordinator*
Rosanne Sodzi	*CESDI Regional Coordinator*
Janet Davis	*CESDI Regional Coordinator*
Pat Finnemore	*Research Health Visitor*
Margaret Griffin	*Research Health Visitor*
Pat Johnson	*Research Health Visitor*
Chris Laws	*Research Midwife*
Rosie McCabe	*Research Midwife*
Sandy Staff	*Research Health Visitor*
Lynda Wood	*Research Health Visitor*
Pam Nadin	*Research Health Visitor*
Charlotte Leach	*Research Assistant*

Yorkshire

Dr Christopher Bacon	*Consultant Paediatrician*
Dr Iain Smith	*Honorary Consultant Child Health*
David Bensley	*Statistician*
Dr Eleanor Allibone	*CESDI Pathologist*
Leslie Anson	*CESDI Regional Coordinator*
Suzanne Page	*Project Administrator*
Janice Peacock	*Assistant CESDI Coordinator*
Lindsay Cansfield	*Research Health Visitor*
Pam Mueller	*Research Health Visitor*
Shirley Stephenson	*Research Health Visitor*
Dawn Taylor	*Research Health Visitor*

Trent

Dr Elizabeth M Taylor	*Medical Advisor*
Professor David Hall	*Medical Advisor*
Dr Valerie Harpin	*Medical Advisor*
Dr Elizabeth Adamson	*Medical Advisor*
Dr Pat McKeever	*Lead Paediatric Pathologist*
Sue Wood	*CESDI Regional Coordinator*
Jayne Bennett	*Administrator for SUDI*

Christine Ahronson	*Research Health Visitor*
Carmel Davitt	*Research Health Visitor*
Lynne Middleton	*Research Health Visitor*
Lorraine Wright	*Research Health Visitor*
Marion Aaron	*Research Health Visitor*
Liz Brown	*Research Health Visitor*
Lynnette Lovelock	*Research Health Visitor*
Ronda Ninkovic	*Research Health Visitor*

Northern

Dr Martin Ward Platt	*Consultant Paediatrician*
Dr Christopher Wright	*Consultant Perinatal Pathologist*
Dr Edmund Hey	*Consultant Paediatrician*
Marjorie Renwick	*CESDI Regional Coordinator*
Marion Malby	*Research Health Visitor*
Kath Brown	*Research Health Visitor*
Jeanette Chatterjee	*Research Health Visitor*

Other Contributors

Dr Shireen Chantler	*Scientific Advisor, Foundation for the Study of Infant Deaths*
Professor Tim Cole	*Professor of Medical Statistics, London*
Dr Jeanine Young	*Research Nurse, Bristol*

FOREWORD

When CESDI was set up in 1992, the National Advisory Body (NAB) decided that the theme of the first programme should be why apparently normal babies which would be expected to thrive did not survive.

Despite the fall in incidence of Sudden Infant Death Syndrome (SIDS), popularly known as 'cot deaths', following the Back to Sleep campaign in 1991, Sudden Unexpected Deaths in Infancy (SUDI) remained the largest single group of deaths in the post-neonatal period. Although these deaths form only a small proportion of all losses in the CESDI age range, they generate considerable public interest and anxiety.

The NAB decided to include in the first CESDI programme confidential enquiries with enhanced pathology into sudden unexpected deaths of babies aged between 7 and 364 days in three NHS regions, South-Western, Yorkshire and Trent, which had appropriate epidemiology and pathology resources. These were accompanied by case studies using four controls and interviews with parents. It was hoped that the SUDI studies would not only identify possible associations and risk factors which might be avoidable or amenable to treatment and make recommendations on professional issues, but that they would also lead to improvements in the methodology of future enquiries.

The studies with which this report is concerned began in February 1993. They were extended in 1995 to cover the former NHS regions of Northern and Wessex, and to gather material which might help the Independent Expert Group, chaired by Lady Limerick, charged with investigating the hypothesis that toxic gases generated by mattress covers might be a cause of SIDS.

The NAB published preliminary results of the first two years of the studies in the 3rd CESDI report. Six key health messages designed to avoid cot deaths were subsequently published in a leaflet of advice to parents. The 5th CESDI report included findings and recommendations relating to SUDI deaths other than SIDS, i.e. the explained deaths, which occurred in the three years of the study.

The NAB always hoped the main results of the three years of the SUDI studies would be brought together in one document. At its final meeting in March 1999, the NAB was pleased to learn that this was in hand and that it would be consulted about the draft report. The NAB is in general agreement with the report's findings and recommendations.

Lady Littler
Chair of the National Advisory Body for CESDI 1992–1999

PREFACE

In the last 20 years the number of infant deaths in the UK has halved. This welcome decrease does not alter the fact that infancy remains the most dangerous period of childhood and that the cause of many deaths remains a mystery. From 1993–1996 all babies dying between the ages of one week and one year, in five English regions were investigated by a multi-disciplinary research team. During the three years, the investigators studied the deaths from nearly half a million live births – a figure close to the total number of babies born in England in one year. They compared the circumstances of each dead infant with four control infants born in the same week. The outcome of the confidential enquiry is one of the most comprehensive scientific paediatric research studies to come from the UK. Much of the great merit of the information stems from its large scale and its contemporary nature. Too much of the quoted information about sudden infant deaths comes from studies which were uncontrolled, of small scale, or relate to earlier times when definition and classification were imprecise, and investigation and assessment very limited. It is good that the detailed new information together with the wide-ranging and thoughtful recommendations are now available in this book.

The recommendations provide a challenge to society, its politicians and its health professionals. There is clear scientific evidence suggesting more appropriate and safer ways of caring for infants and for organising their nursing and medical care. Whilst it is true that impact of social circumstances, particularly in relation to unexplained deaths – 'Sudden Infant Death Syndrome' – is very large (an infant of a young mother who smokes and is on income support is 40 times more likely to die than that of a 35-year-old, non-smoking mother in a home where she or her partner have a regular income), there are still many practical steps that can be implemented to safeguard children in *all* homes. The knowledge needs to be spread and health professionals should be in the vanguard of that propaganda.

The number of deaths classified as SIDS continues to fall, but it is a matter of concern and perhaps anger that both health workers and the public readily accept a situation in which the deaths of so many infants remain poorly investigated, poorly understood and rather casually categorised and dismissed as 'cases of SIDS'. Unless the cause of a problem is understood there is little chance of prevention or cure. The studies in this book make clear the benefits of a more rigorous investigation of infants deaths involving: assessment of the death scene; review of the circumstances and previous medical history of the child; and a detailed post-mortem by an experienced pathologist. A multi-disciplinary review of those findings will identify the probable cause in many cases, and contributory factors in many more.

Comprehensive assessment of all sudden infant deaths in the UK could be achieved with a relatively small increase in resource. Such assessment is both feasible and necessary – for parents who want to know why their child died; for children who are dying needlessly; and for their brothers and sisters who may remain at risk of death or disability unless the cause of the infant death is identified.

For the thousands of parents who provided information for this research, the book represents a fitting memorial to the infants who died. However, this book is a sign post, not a tombstone. It tells us how we, whether as parents, politicians or health workers, should alter our ways to provide a safer and healthier future for children.

Professor Sir Roy Meadow
BM BCh, MA, FRCP, FRCPE, FRCPH, DCH, DRCOG
Past President, Royal College of Paediatrics and Child Health
Emeritus Professor of Paediatrics and Child Health, University of Leeds

ACKNOWLEDGEMENTS

These studies were supported by research grants from the National Advisory Body for CESDI, the Foundation for the Study of Infant Deaths and the Department of Health.

We wish to express our thanks and appreciation to the families of the infants who died, the families of the control infants, and the health care professionals from many disciplines, whose support, cooperation, and help made this study possible. The willingness of the families to share with us many aspects of their lives, in the hope that we would be able to help prevent other babies dying in this way was an inspiration to all who worked on the project.

 giving babies the chance of a lifetime

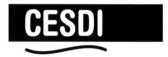

Chapter 1
_____

INTRODUCTION

Chris Bacon

Deaths in infancy

When most of the population live in poverty a high proportion of babies die in the first year of life from malnutrition and infection. This was the case in Britain in past centuries, as it still is in the poorest parts of the world today. As the standard of living rises infant mortality falls, so that now in advanced countries fewer than 10 out of every 1,000 babies born will die before their first birthday. Figure 1.1 shows the present distribution of the main causes of infant death in England and Wales. For the largest categories, immaturity and congenital abnormality, death usually occurs in the first week of life. In other categories of known cause such as infection, malignancy, metabolic disease and accidents, deaths are spread over the first 12 months of life.

Figure 1.1   Distribution of main categories of infant death in England and Wales in 1997

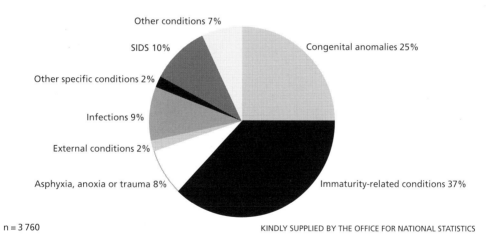

n = 3 760   KINDLY SUPPLIED BY THE OFFICE FOR NATIONAL STATISTICS

Sudden unexpected deaths

There is also a substantial group where death comes suddenly and unexpectedly, as it were out of the blue. In some of these unexpected deaths a cause may subsequently be determined, either by scrutiny of the circumstances or by autopsy. For example, it may become apparent that the baby died from accidental suffocation or from an undiagnosed heart defect: the death can then be allocated to the appropriate specific category. However, more often, in about four unexpected deaths out of five, no clear cause can be found: the death remains unexplained and may then be categorised as sudden infant death syndrome (SIDS). SIDS comprises the largest category of deaths occurring in England and Wales between the ages of one month and one year – that is, post-neonatal infant deaths (Figure 1.2).

Sudden infant death syndrome

Reports of babies dying unexpectedly go far back in western literature, an early and oft-quoted example being the death of the baby that prompted the legendary judgement of King Solomon [1] – although this death was not typical of SIDS in that it occurred in the first week of life. However, it is only in the last 50 years or so, during which time such deaths have emerged as a significant proportion of total infant mortality, that they have become a focus of medical interest and research. In 1969, the American pathologist Beckwith [2] formulated the definition of SIDS that is still current: 'the sudden death of a baby that is unexpected by history and in whom a thorough necropsy examination fails to demonstrate an adequate cause of death'. The term SIDS was introduced partly for humanitarian reasons, being intended as a recognised category of natural death that carried no implication of blame for bereaved parents. Subsequent proposals to elaborate on the diagnostic criteria for SIDS by requiring that the search for a cause of death should include, in addition to history and autopsy, an investigation of the scene or circumstances of the death [3,4], have been widely supported but not yet universally adopted.

In 1971 SIDS became registrable as a cause of death in England and Wales, and it was then possible for the Office for National Statistics (formerly the Office of Population, Censuses and Surveys) to publish annual totals of registrations. There is no way of determining the incidence of SIDS prior to that date, because deaths that would thereafter come to be categorised as SIDS had been attributed to another cause, usually respiratory infection. For the first few years after 1971 the figures are misleading because it took time for the new registration to become established.

Figure 1.2   Distribution of main categories of post-neonatal infant death in England and Wales in 1997

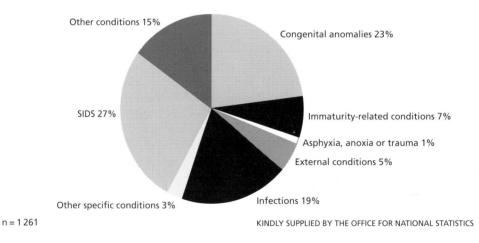

Other conditions 15%

Congenital anomalies 23%

SIDS 27%

Immaturity-related conditions 7%

Asphyxia, anoxia or trauma 1%

External conditions 5%

Other specific conditions 3%

Infections 19%

n = 1 261

KINDLY SUPPLIED BY THE OFFICE FOR NATIONAL STATISTICS

Inconsistencies in the definition of SIDS

The definition of SIDS allows considerable scope for inconsistency, depending as it does upon the pathologist's thoroughness in the autopsy and upon his or her interpretation of the findings. For example, in one area infant autopsies may usually be carried out by a specialist pathologist who will routinely carry out a full range of investigations, including detailed histological and microbiological studies, while in another area autopsies may be limited to macroscopic inspection and hence less likely to detect covert disease. Furthermore, two pathologists making the same findings may not agree on whether they constitute an adequate explanation for death: for example, if there are signs of respiratory infection one might give this as the cause of death, while the other might regard it as coincidental and classify the death as SIDS. In addition, pathologists and coroners may vary in their readiness to accept SIDS as a registered cause of death, sometimes preferring terms such as 'cardio-respiratory failure' or 'unascertained'. These variations may give rise to inconsistency in the reporting of SIDS in different places in the United Kingdom. Inevitably, there will be similar inconsistencies between different countries, so that international comparisons of SIDS rates should be interpreted with caution. However, pathologists are now working towards international consensus on a standard protocol for autopsies following unexpected infant death [5].

The classification and terminology of sudden infant death

Besides these problems of definition, there are other possible sources of confusion in the classification and terminology of sudden infant death.

Firstly, three different age ranges may be quoted: birth to 52 weeks ('infant deaths'), 1– 52 weeks ('post-perinatal deaths') or 4–52 weeks ('post-neonatal deaths'). The study that forms the subject of this report deals with post-perinatal deaths.

Secondly, the categories used for official statistics do not exactly correspond with medical definitions. In its annual figures for causes of infant deaths in England and Wales the Office for National Statistics (ONS) currently follows the codes laid down in the ninth revision of the International Classification of Diseases (ICD). The ONS allocates to ICD code 798.0, entitled 'Sudden infant death syndrome', those deaths for which SIDS or the equivalent is the sole cause entered on the death certificate. These cases are all likely to have met the Beckwith criteria for SIDS. The ONS also publishes figures for sudden infant death under another broader heading that includes, in addition to the deaths coded under ICD 798.0, about 30–40 further deaths a year in which the death certificate gives another condition, such as respiratory infection, as well as sudden infant death or an equivalent term. International guidelines require the selection of the more precise condition for the purpose of ICD coding. In respect of medical definition, however, two different categories may be found among these deaths with dual entries on the certificate. In some, the specific condition will not have been regarded as an adequate cause of death and the Beckwith criteria for SIDS will have been met, despite allocation to the more specific ICD code; in others the specific condition will have been identified as an adequate underlying cause, despite the mention of sudden infant death on the certificate. A further complication is that not all sudden deaths that have been explained at autopsy are included under this broad ONS heading, because the ONS can identify only those where the term 'sudden' or 'cot death' is entered on the certificate. These imprecisions arise from variations in the reporting practices of pathologists and coroners. As a result, it is not possible to determine from current ONS figures precise totals either for all sudden infant deaths or for those that meet the Beckwith criteria for SIDS.

Thirdly, the exact meaning of the lay term 'cot death' ('crib death' in the USA), which was coined by Barratt in 1954 [6], is still the subject of debate [7,8]. Some people restrict it to deaths meeting the Beckwith criteria for SIDS, while others give it the wider meaning of any infant death that occurs suddenly and unexpectedly, regardless of whether or not a cause is subsequently determined. Besides this imprecision, the term can be misleading by its implication that death always occurs in the cot, which, although usual, is not invariable.

Finally, the grouping for the deaths in the Confidential Enquiry for Stillbirths and Deaths in Infancy (CESDI) study, which was given the acronym SUDI (sudden unexpected deaths in infancy), does not correspond with any single ICD or ONS classification, and includes various other unexpected deaths as well as SIDS. The criteria for inclusion are given in Chapter 2, while the reasons for the choice of this wider definition are explained below ('CESDI study of SUDI').

Definition by exclusion

Several of the problems described above arise from the fact that SIDS, although listed by the ICD and ONS among 'underlying causes of death', is not a positive diagnosis for a specific condition but rather a categorisation of exclusion. It is generally accepted that there is no unitary explanation for SIDS, but rather that it comprises a heterogeneous collection of deaths arising from several different causes, acting singly or in combination. Although research has so far left many questions unanswered, it is theoretically possible that the day will come when our understanding of all the specific mechanisms of infant death and our techniques for identifying them have improved to the point that categorisation as SIDS is no longer needed.

Epidemiology of SIDS

Studies in many countries over the past 30 years have painted a similar epidemiological profile of families in which SIDS most typically occurs [9]. Most at risk are babies who are premature, of low birth weight or from multiple births; whose mothers are young, poorly educated, live in poor conditions, smoke and leave little interval between pregnancies; whose fathers are absent or unemployed. Deaths are uncommon in the first month of life, rise abruptly to a peak at about 10 weeks and then fall more gradually, becoming infrequent after six months and very unusual beyond a year. Deaths usually occur during the night and are more frequent in the winter months. Boys are more vulnerable than girls, and some ethnic groups are less vulnerable than others.

Incidence of SIDS in England and Wales

Figure 1.3 shows the post-neonatal rates for SIDS (ICD 798.0, or ICD 795 prior to the revision of ICD in 1979) and various other categories of death in infancy reported by the ONS for England and Wales since 1971. The apparently low rates for SIDS in the earlier years reflect the time it took for this designation to achieve general acceptance as a registrable cause of death. The rate had levelled out at about 1.7 per 1,000 live births in the early 1980s, but then began to rise again to a peak of 2.0 per 1,000 in 1988, when 1,390 post-neonatal deaths coded as SIDS occurred in a single year. At the same time, certain other European countries were reporting rates appreciably lower than those of England and Wales.

The origins of CESDI

The rise in the rate for SIDS and for infant mortality as a whole in 1986 was in part responsible for the eventual setting up of the Confidential Enquiry for Stillbirths and Deaths in Infancy (CESDI) some six years later. In 1988, the Social Services Committee of the House of Commons expressed its concern about this rise [10] and urged that immediate steps should be taken to improve the situation. The Government responded with various recommendations [11], including the proposals that there should be further research into infant deaths, particularly those attributed to SIDS, and that all unexplained infant deaths should be routinely examined by a regional confidential enquiry. A working group was then set up by the Chief Medical Officer to consider the feasibility of these proposals, and its report of 1990 [12] set out the basis for the establishment of a national confidential enquiry into all stillbirths and deaths in infancy. The National Advisory Body for CESDI was established the following year, and the first enquiries under its auspices began in early 1993.

Figure 1.3 Cumulative post-neonatal deaths by selected causes, England and Wales, 1971–1997

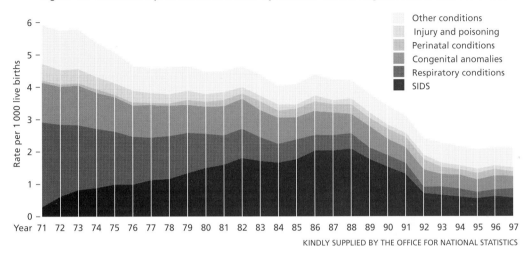

KINDLY SUPPLIED BY THE OFFICE FOR NATIONAL STATISTICS

Meanwhile, between 1988 and 1993 there had been a marked fall in the incidence of SIDS in England and Wales, so that the high rate that had played a part in instigating the establishment of CESDI had more than halved by the time the enquiry got under way. The reasons for this fall are not fully understood, but it is thought to have resulted largely from a change in practice in the way babies were put down to sleep. In the late 1980s and early 1990s evidence was emerging that prone sleeping brought a higher risk of SIDS, and in 1991 national campaigns were started to encourage mothers to put their babies on their backs or their sides [13–17]. This welcome improvement in the SIDS rate did not diminish the need for CESDI, whose remit covered the whole range of deaths from 20 weeks of gestation to the end of the first year of life. It was felt that an enquiry into SIDS was still appropriate because this remained the single largest category of deaths in the post-neonatal period and was the subject of much public anxiety. In addition, it was thought opportune to investigate whether there had been a change in the epidemiological pattern of SIDS after the intervention on sleeping position had taken effect, in the hope of finding further factors that might be amenable to intervention.

CESDI study of SUDI

For these reasons, the National Advisory Body selected sudden deaths in infancy to be the subject of one of the first detailed studies undertaken when CESDI got under way in the beginning of 1993. The broader category of SUDI rather than SIDS was chosen because it is often not possible to distinguish between SIDS and other unexpected deaths until the full autopsy results become available, which may not be for some weeks after the death, and even then the distinction may not be clear-cut. In addition, it was expected that health professionals would more often have been involved in the care of babies whose deaths were explained, so that enquiry into these would be more likely to yield lessons in professional audit and consequent improvements in service.

References

1. *Holy Bible*. I Kings, chapter 3, verses 16–28.

2. Beckwith, JB. 'Discussion of terminology and definition of the sudden infant death syndrome', in Bergman, JB and Ray, CG (eds) *Proceedings of the Second International Conference on Causes of Sudden Death in Infants*. Seattle: University of Washington Press, 1970: 14–22.

3. Willinger, M, James, LS and Catz, C. 'Defining the sudden infant death syndrome (SIDS): deliberations of an expert panel convened by the National Institute of Child Health and Human Development', *Pediatric Pathology*, 1991; 11: 677–84.

4. Rognum, TO and Willinger, M. 'The story of the "Stavanger definition"' in Rognum, TO (ed.) *Sudden Infant Death Syndrome: New Trends in the Nineties*. Oslo: Scandinavian University Press, 1995: 21–5.

5. Krous, HF. 'The international standardised autopsy protocol for sudden unexpected infant death' in Rognum TO (ed.) *Sudden Infant Death Syndrome: New Trends in the Nineties*. Oslo: Scandinavian University Press, 1995: 81–95.

6. Barratt, AM. 'Sudden death in infancy' in Gairdner, D (ed.) *Recent Advances in Paediatrics*. Churchill Livingstone, 1954: 301–20.

7. Limerick, SR and Gardner, A. 'What counts as cot death?', *British Medical Journal*, 1992; 304: 1176.

8. Gordon, RR. 'What counts as cot death?', *British Medical Journal*, 1992; 304: 1508.

9. Golding, J, Limerick, S and Macfarlane, A. *Sudden Infant Death: Patterns, Puzzles and Problems*. Shepton Mallet: Open Books, 1985: 22–102.

10. House of Commons Social Services Committee. *Perinatal, Neonatal and Infant Mortality*, session 1988–89, first report. London: HMSO, 1988.

11. Department of Health. *Perinatal, Neonatal and Infant Mortality*, Government reply to the first report from the Social Services Committee. London: HMSO, 1989.

12. Department of Health. *Confidential Enquiry into Stillbirths and Deaths in Infancy*, report of a working group set up by the Chief Medical Officer. London: DoH, 1990.

13. Fleming, PJ, Gilbert, RE, Azaz, Y, Berry, PJ, Rudd, PT, Stewart, A and Hall, E. 'The interaction between bedding and sleeping position in sudden infant death syndrome: a population-based case-control study', *British Medical Journal*, 1990; 301: 85–9.

14. Wigfield, RE, Fleming, PJ, Berry, PJ, Rudd, PT and Golding, J. 'Can the fall in Avon's sudden infant death rate be explained by the observed sleeping position changes?', *British Medical Journal*, 1992; 304: 282–3.

15. Foundation for the Study of Infant Deaths. *Reduce the Risks of Cot Death* (leaflet). FSID, 1991.

16. Department of Health. *Back to sleep: reducing the risk of cot death* (leaflet). London: DoH, 1991.

17. Stewart, AJ, Mitchell, EA, Tipene Leach, D and Fleming, PJ. 'Lessons from the New Zealand and United Kingdom Cot Death Campaigns', *Acta Paediatr. Scand.*,1993; supplement 389: 119–23.

Chapter 2

DESIGN OF THE SUDI STUDY

Chris Bacon and Peter Fleming

Populations and periods of study

The SUDI study began in two former National Health Service (NHS) regions, South-Western and Yorkshire, on 1 February 1993. A third region, Trent, joined the study in September 1993, and two more regions, Northern and Wessex, joined in April 1995. Case enrolment ceased in all regions on 31 March 1996. The total population of the five regions was 17.7 million, and the total number of births, allowing for the different periods of study in each region, was just under half a million. This compares with a total of about 650,000 births a year in England and Wales during the study period.

It had originally been intended that the SUDI study should take place in three regions and last for two years. However, an extension was agreed so the study could be used to collect data and material that might assist the Limerick Committee, which in 1994 began to investigate the hypothesis that toxic gases generated from mattress covers might be a cause of SIDS [1]. An additional advantage of this extension, which was funded partly by the Foundation for the Study of Infant Deaths, was that the extra numbers helped to reinforce the power of the study as a whole, which the declining incidence of SIDS had caused to fall below that originally intended.

Objectives

The main objectives of the SUDI study as given in the Third Annual Report for CESDI [2] were as follows:

- to identify possible risk factors and associations for sudden unexpected infant deaths, and in particular those factors that might be avoidable or amenable to intervention;
- to audit the performance of health care professionals with regard to babies who had died, and to make recommendations on professional issues;
- to determine which pathological investigatons are most important following the sudden unexpected death of an infant;
- to evaluate methods for enquiring into sudden unexpected deaths in infancy, including the role of parental interviews, the efficacy of confidential enquiries, the use of controls and the contribution of various systems for classifying deaths and the factors relating to them;
- to identify areas requiring further study.

In addition, it became apparent, after the marked decline in infant deaths following the intervention on sleeping position, that a further important objective would be to delineate the new epidemiological profile of SIDS that had emerged.

Definition of SUDI

The age range for the SUDI study was babies who died between seven and 365 completed days of life (i.e. post-perinatal infant deaths). The criteria for inclusion were:

- deaths that were unexpected, and unexplained at autopsy (i.e. those meeting the criteria for SIDS);

- deaths occurring in the course of an acute illness that was not recognised by carers and/or by health professionals as potentially life-threatening;

- deaths occurring in the course of a sudden acute illness of less than 24 hours' duration in a previously healthy infant, or a death that occurred after this if intensive care had been instituted within 24 hours of the onset of the illness;

- deaths arising from a pre-existing condition that had not been previously recognised by health professionals;

- deaths resulting from any form of accident, trauma or poisoning.

Components of SUDI study

The SUDI study was designed to have three components:

- a case-control study;
- additional pathology investigations;
- confidential enquiries by regional assessment panels (on index cases only).

The same index cases served as subjects both for the case-control study and for the confidential enquiry, these two components of the study sharing a common structure for the purpose of administration and data collection. Such an arrangement is thought to be unique for a study on this scale. The three components of the study were linked in that the pathology investigations helped to inform the confidential enquiries, whose judgements determined the category of death used for the case-control study.

Administrative structure

The administrative structure for the SUDI study, as for other parts of the CESDI programme, was in three tiers. At national level the National Advisory Body, supported by the secretariat, was responsible for the institution and general oversight of the project. Each participating region had its own coordinator and clinical advisers, who met together regularly to ensure consistency of approach. Each region appointed its own research interviewers, who were ex-health visitors and had standard additional training. At district level there was a further network of coordinators, usually paediatricians or senior nurses, who were responsible for the ascertainment of cases. Ethical approval was obtained from the ethics committee of each district individually.

Protocol and questionnaire

The original protocol for the SUDI studies was published in the First Annual Report for CESDI [3]. Minor modifications were subsequently made in the light of experience, and in the third year additional procedures were incorporated to allow examination of the hypothesis that toxic gases might be produced from mattress covers (see Chapter 3). The parental questionnaire, which can be viewed on the website at http://www.official-documents.co.uk/document/doh/cesdi/enquiry.htm, covered more than 600 fields, including demographic and social data; the medical history of the baby and other family members; use of cigarettes, alcohol and drugs; the precise sleeping arrangements for the baby, with regard both to the family's usual practices and to the period when the baby died; and full details of the events preceding and the circumstances surrounding the death.

Ascertainment of cases

Reporting networks were set up in every participating district or trust, using multiple sources, including general practitioners, midwives, health visitors, paediatricians, neonatal units, emergency departments, ambulance control, pathologists, mortuary attendants, coroners and coroners' officers, and parent support groups. Deaths were reported as soon as possible to the district coordinator, who would then inform the appropriate research interviewer, putting her in touch with the health visitor for the family. The multiplicity of sources ensured that ascertainment was as complete as possible, while any duplication in reporting could be readily resolved by the coordinator. In most cases the research interviewer was informed within 24 hours of the death.

Parental interviews

The research interviewers visited each bereaved family twice. On the first visit, which was arranged through the family's health visitor and usually took place within five days of the death, after obtaining informed consent interviewers took a standardised semi-structured history, including a narrative account of events leading up to the baby's death. The interviewer would also answer questions and offer to arrange support and counselling as appropriate, this aspect of their role being emphasised in training. On the second visit, a few days later and usually within two weeks of the death, they completed the bulk of the questionnaire from the answers given by the family. The remaining items were obtained from medical and nursing records.

Excluded data

Families were not interviewed when it was suspected at an early stage that death had resulted from non-accidental injury and the police were likely to be involved. However, in these cases, and in those where parental consent to interview was withheld, information was collected from public records such as birth and death certificates. In addition, research interviewers had discretion to exclude items in the questionnaire that were clearly not relevant to a particular case (for example, details of the last sleeping arrangements for a baby who had died in a car accident).

Controls

The health visitor for the baby who had died was asked to identify as controls four babies on her list born within two weeks of the index baby, two older and two younger. If her list did not include four babies who met these requirements she drew from the list of her nearest colleague. In the few instances where the family thus identified was not available or did not wish to participate, or when inclusion was thought inappropriate, for example, because of recent bereavement, then the family with the baby next closest in age was substituted. The interviewer visited each control family within a week of the death to collect the same data as for the index case. A period of sleep, termed the 'reference sleep', was identified in the life of the control baby in the 24 hours before the interview that corresponded to the time of day in which the index baby had died, with emphasis on the index parents' view of whether it had been a night or daytime sleep. Data were collected for this reference sleep equivalent to those collected for the index baby.

Autopsies

Since all deaths were unexpected, an autopsy was routinely required by the coroner, who might instruct a paediatric pathologist, a forensic pathologist or a general pathologist according to the circumstances. All pathologists carrying out autopsies on SUDI cases were asked to include in their examination the investigations recommended by the Royal College of Pathologists and outlined in the First Annual Report for CESDI [4]. Appropriate extra funding was made available for this purpose. Prior to the autopsy, parents were given a copy of the leaflet *Guide to the post-mortem examination*, which explains the purpose and procedure for autopsies [5]. This leaflet was produced by the Stillbirth and Neonatal Death Society, the Foundation for the Study of Infant Deaths, the Royal College of Pathologists and CESDI, and is available in several languages.

Local case discussion

The protocol for the SUDI study required that a local case discussion should be held after each relevant death, as has been standard practice in many areas. The discussion was held as soon as the full autopsy results were available (usually after about six weeks), and normally took place in the general practitioner's surgery. Intended participants included the research interviewer, the general practitioner, the midwife (when relevant), the health visitor, the pathologist and a paediatrician. The main objectives of this discussion were to review the circumstances of the death and the autopsy findings, to identify any avoidable factors or lessons for the future, and to plan continuing support for the family. A summary of the discussion was recorded on a standard pro forma, including any information additional to or at variance with that obtained at the parental interview.

Regional panels for confidential enquiry

All cases for which sufficient information was available were assessed by regional panels. These panels could not be held until at least two months after the death had occurred because of the need to await reports on post-mortem histology and from the local case discussion. Confidentiality was maintained by anonymising all papers, and by ensuring that no panel member had prior knowledge of the case in question. To improve consistency, the chairs for the panels in each region were permanent, while other panel members were drawn from a small pool of experienced practitioners in each specialty. Panel membership always included a general practitioner, a health visitor, an obstetrician or a midwife, a paediatrician, a paediatric pathologist and a public health doctor. The research interviewer was not present at the panel but contributed to the documentation.

Documentation

Panel members were provided in advance with copies of all available documents for each case, including:

■   the questionnaire completed by the research interviewer;

■   the obstetric and midwifery notes;

■   the general practitioner's notes;

- the health visitor's notes;
- paediatric and paediatric nursing records;
- records from emergency departments;
- the autopsy report;
- the summary of the local case discussion;
- ambulance records.

In many instances, there had been no attendance at a paediatric or emergency department. In addition, many general practitioners were unwilling to make their notes available.

Procedure for regional panels

Panels were required to arrive at a consensus view of the following:

- a brief summary of the case;
- classification of the death by the Sheffield and Avon systems [6,7];
- identification and assessment of notable factors by the Exeter system [8];
- other points of interest, particularly those relating to the process of the enquiry.

Classification by the Avon system

The Avon system [7] of classification gives a measure of the extent to which the autopsy findings provide an explanation for a baby's death. After assessment of all available clinical and pathological information, deaths are placed in one of three broad categories:

I. no significant findings;

II. findings that may have contributed to ill health and possibly to death;

III. findings that provide a full explanation for death.

For the purposes of the study, deaths that the regional panels placed in groups I and II were categorised as SIDS, while those in group III were categorised as explained deaths. This categorisation by the regional panel did not necessarily correspond with the assessment made by the original pathologist and thus with the registered cause of death. Such differences of opinion were uncommon, and usually arose from the judgement as to whether the autopsy findings constituted a full explanation for the death. Panels would be guided on this point by their paediatric pathologist, who in addition to seeing the full autopsy report was also able to review the histological sections.

Identification of sub-optimal care

Panels were required to identify notable factors relating to each case following the Exeter system, as described in a previous report [8]. These factors included instances of sub-optimal care by professionals or by carers that in the opinion of the panel probably or possibly contributed to the death of the baby.

Statistical methodology for the univariate and multivariate analysis

Odds ratios (ORs), 95% confidence intervals (CIs) and p-values for the univariate and multivariate analyses were calculated taking into account the matching using conditional logistic regression (see

Chapter 3, p.72) in the statistical package SAS [9]. The age of the control infant was taken as the age at reference sleep in the 24 hours prior to interview. Because of the time required to arrange four control interviews, the control infants were approximately 10 days older than the index infants. The variable for infant age was therefore included in all univariate and multivariate analyses. Models were constructed using the stepwise procedure [10] for variables significant at the 5% level in the univariate analysis.

Percentages were quoted to one decimal place rounding error for the summation of total percentage will be no more than 0.1%.

Data that were not normally distributed were described using medians and inter-quartile ranges (IQRs).

References

1. Richardson, BA. 'Sudden infant death syndrome: a possible primary cause', *Journal of the Forensic Science Society*, 1994; 34: 199–204.

2. Department of Health. *Confidential Enquiry into Stillbirths and Deaths in Infancy: Third Annual Report*. London: DoH, 1996: para 5.2.

3. Department of Health. *Confidential Enquiry into Stillbirths and Deaths in Infancy: First Annual Report*. London: HMSO, 1993: appendix F.

4. Department of Health. *Confidential Enquiry into Stillbirths and Deaths in Infancy: First Annual Report*. London: HMSO, 1993: appendices E and F.

5. Department of Health. *Guide to the post-mortem examination: brief notes for parents and families who have lost a baby in pregnancy or early infancy*. London: DoH, 1993.

6. Taylor, EM and Emery, JL. 'Categories of preventable unexpected infant deaths', *Archives of Disease in Childhood*, 1990; 65: 535–9.

7. Gilbert, R, Rudd, P, Berry,PJ, Fleming, PJ, Hall, E, White, DG, Oreffo, VO, James, P and Evans, JA. 'Combined effect of infection and heavy wrapping on the risk of sudden infant death', *Archives of Disease in Childhood*, 1992; 67: 171–7.

8. Department of Health. *Confidential Enquiry into Stillbirths and Deaths in Infancy: Third Annual Report*. London: DoH, 1996: chapter 7.

9. SAS Institute Inc. *SAS Technical Report P-229, SAS/STAT Software: Changes and Enhancements, Release 6.07*, Cary, NC: SAS Institute Inc., 1992.

10. Kleinbaum, DG. *Logistic regression: a self-learning text* (Statistics in the Health Sciences series). New York: Springer Verlag, 1994.

Chapter 3

THE CASE-CONTROL STUDY: RESULTS AND DISCUSSION

Peter Fleming, Peter Blair, Martin Ward Platt, Iain Smith and Shireen Chantler

ASCERTAINMENT

Study area

The study was conducted between February 1993 and March 1996 in five former health regions of England, during the periods shown in Table 3.1.

Table 3.1 Study period for each health region

Region	Start Date	Finish Date
Northern	1 April 1995	31 March 1996
South-West	1 February 1993	31 March 1996
Trent	1 September 1993	31 March 1996
Wessex	1 April 1995	31 March 1996
Yorkshire	1 February 1993	31 March 1996

Deaths during February and March 1995 were excluded from the study to provide time to expand the study base to include two more health regions and organise the collection of infant mattresses, tissue and hair samples and household dust for the third year of the study.

The population for the five regions (using ONS mid-1995 estimates) was 17.7 million and the total number of live births in the study regions during the study period was over 470,000. This compares with a total of approximately 650,000 births a year in England and Wales during the study period.

Classification of cases and regional breakdown

During the study period, a total of 456 cases of sudden unexpected death in infancy (SUDI) aged between one week and one year were identified, of which 93 were later fully explained and 363 were classified as sudden infant death syndrome (SIDS) by the Avon clinico-pathological classification system [1], as described in Chapter 2. For some of the cases (e.g. those suspected of non-accidental injury) no confidential enquiry meeting was held. For these deaths, the findings at the local case discussion were used to determine the cause of death. The number of deaths by classification category are shown in Table 3.2.

Table 3.2 Number of deaths in each group, using the Avon classification system

Avon Classification	n = 456	%
I No abnormal findings		
IA No abnormal findings	70	15.4
IB Non-contributory findings	109	23.9
I A/B (Classed as I but unsure of subgroup)	10	2.2
II Associated findings		
IIA Possibly contributory associated findings	113	24.8
IIB Extensive findings, but not complete explanation	44	9.6
II A/B (Classed as II but unsure of subgroup)	10	2.2
I or II (No classification given)	7	1.5
Total of I and II (i.e. SIDS)	363	79.6
III Fully explained death	93	20.4

Note: Percentages are presented to one decimal place which can lead to a 0.1% rounding error for the total percentage for this and subsequent tables.

Deaths in groups I and II thus met the definition of SIDS: the death of an infant which was unexpected by history, and which remained unexplained after a full post-mortem examination,* an investigation of the circumstances of death and a detailed review of the medical and social history by a multidisciplinary regional panel [2]. Deaths in group III were those for which the regional panel found a complete explanation of the death, from post-mortem findings, the circumstances of death, or both.

The number of deaths by region are shown in Table 3.3.

Table 3.3 Regional breakdown of all identified cases

Region	All SUDI		Explained deaths		SIDS		SIDS rate (95% CI)*	Number of live births[†]
	n	%	n	%	n	%		
Northern	34	7.5	10	10.8	24	6.6	0.70 (0.42–0.99)	34 103
South West	111	24.3	17	18.3	94	25.9	0.81 (0.65–0.97)	116 263
Trent	143	31.4	30	32.3	113	31.1	0.79 (0.65–0.94)	142 646
Wessex	21	4.6	4	4.3	17	4.7	0.45 (0.24–0.67)	37 510
Yorkshire	147	32.2	32	34.4	115	31.7	0.81 (0.66–0.96)	142 301
Total	456		93		363		0.77 (0.69–0.85)	472 823

* CI = confidence interval per 1,000 live births

† Using number of live births for each region from January to December: 1993–1995 (ONS) for the South-West, Trent and Yorkshire – approximating Trent Region's contribution in the first year of the study as 5/12ths of the 1993 live births for that region; 1995 (ONS) for Northern and Wessex

The proportion of explained SUDI ranged from 15–29% amongst the study regions. The SIDS rates were very similar for four regions, approximately eight deaths per 10,000 live births, with a lower rate, four or five deaths per 10,000 live births, in Wessex.

---

* Information on the protocol for the post-mortem, together with a detailed audit of the examinations actually carried out and an assessment of the value of specific investigations, is given in Chapter 4.

Completeness of notification of deaths

Careful cross-checking of death notifications received by the SUDI offices with those received by the ONS and the registrars' offices, two years after the end of the study period, has identified a total of eight deaths of infants normally resident within the study regions during the study time period that were not notified to the SUDI research teams. These included deaths that occurred in other parts of the country and deaths subject to police investigation. Overall ascertainment of eligible infant deaths was thus 98.3%.

Time to notification and interview

The time from the discovery of the death to notification was recorded accurately for the third study year; 63% were reported to the regional survey offices within 24 hours, and the median time was 14 hours (interquartile range: 3–47 hours).

For the three-year study period, the median interval between discovery of death to the first interview of index parents was four days (interquartile range: 2–10 days), and from first to second interview was seven days (interquartile range: 5–10 days). Over 90% of the control families were interviewed within 12 days of the index death.

Case ascertainment

The families of 328 of the 363 SIDS cases were interviewed. Of the 35 families not interviewed, four were subject to police investigation, seven could not be traced (four moved out of the region and three out of the country), and 24 families did not wish to participate (93.4% consent rate). Epidemiological data available from public records (sex, place of birth, age of baby and parents, time of death, place of death, certified cause of death) were collected on all deaths. Three of the 328 SIDS families interviewed did not live in the study regions and controls were therefore not chosen. The three-year analysis thus concerns 325 SIDS infants.

Of the 93 explained deaths, 74 families were interviewed. Of the 19 families not interviewed, 10 were subject to police investigation; two families could not be traced, one mother was mentally ill and six families did not wish to participate (93.5% consent rate). For two of the 74 families interviewed, controls were not found in the required time period. Hence, the three year analysis concerns 72 explained SUDI deaths.

Control ascertainment

Controls for six families of the total of 456 SUDI were not sought, because they normally lived outside the study regions or because of police involvement. Of the 1,800 controls initially selected, 134 (7.4%) proved unsuitable but were immediately replaced. Of these, 44 parents refused to participate (2.4%), 49 were not contactable after at least two attempts, and 41 were considered unsuitable by their health visitor, mainly because of recent bereavement or illness. In two instances, control families for an explained SUDI death were not found in the required time period so that ascertainment of controls was 99.9%. A full set of four controls per case was thus obtained for the 325 SIDS and 72 explained SUDI cases included in the analysis.

Matching

Age matching of controls was based upon date of birth, but for data analysis age was calculated for index infants from birth to death and for controls from birth to date of interview. Of the controls, 65.8% were matched to within two weeks of the birth of the index baby, and 91.2% within one month. The median age difference between the two groups was 11 days, the control babies being older than the index babies because of the delay to arrange the four control interviews after the death. To accommodate this, age was used as a mandatory variable for all univariate and multivariate models.

Control families were taken from the case load listing of the index health visitor, and were thus partially matched by locality. This had the advantage of immediate access to control families and, particularly amongst the more socially deprived groups, an introduction by a known health care professional (the family's health visitor) facilitated the acceptance of the research interviewer. A potential disadvantage of this selection process was of partial matching by socio-economic status.

Figure 3.1 Comparison of occupational classification of mothers

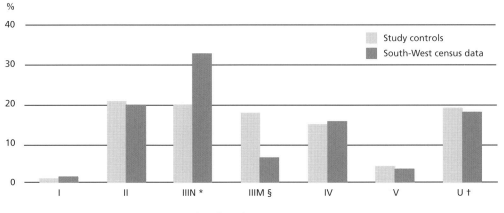

N = 1 588 control mothers and 69 841 mothers from the census
* N = non-manual § M = manual † U = unemployed

In order to ascertain whether there was a systematic distortion of socio-economic status amongst the control families as a result of the selection process, we have compared the socio-economic classification of the control families with data obtained from the 1991 National Census. National data relating specifically to mothers with children under one year of age are not available, but Dr Deborah Baker has used the Census data to analyse the socio-economic status of such mothers in the South-West Region. Figure 3.1 compares the maternal occupation of the control mothers in the SUDI study with that of mothers in the South-West Region. Comparison of the socio-economic status of the study control mothers from the South-West with mothers from the other four regions covered by the study revealed no systematic differences. The population from the whole study was therefore used in this comparison in order to ensure that there were sufficient mothers in each socio-economic group.

There is a difference in the non-manual and manual occupations in the third stratum, but when IIIN and IIIM are combined the overall proportions are very similar (38.5% study controls vs. 40.2% mothers in the Census). Hence, the socio-economic breakdown of control mothers in this study is not different from the generality of mothers in the South-West Region who have a baby under one year old.

EXPLAINED SUDI

Unless otherwise stated, this analysis uses the data from 72 explained SUDI infants and their 288 matched controls.

Inclusion criteria

'Explained SUDI' were those sudden, unexpected deaths for which the regional panels identified a cause of death which they deemed sufficient to constitute a full explanation, and which were thus classified under group III of the Avon classification.

The 'explained SUDI' group thus included:

- those deaths occurring in the course of a sudden acute illness that was not recognised by parents or carers as potentially life-threatening, and may thus not have been brought to the attention of health care professionals;

- those deaths occurring in the course of a sudden acute illness that was not recognised by health care professionals as potentially life-threatening;

- those occurring in the course of a sudden acute illness of less than 24 hours' duration in a previously healthy baby (plus those occurring after the institution of life support in the first 24 hours);

- those arising from a pre-existing condition that had not been previously recognised by health care professionals;

- those arising from any form of accident, trauma or poisoning.

These deaths, and their matched controls, have been considered separately in the analysis from the deaths classified as SIDS.

Causes of death

Table 3.4 gives the causes of death, under broad headings, for the 93 explained SUDI.

Table 3.4   Avon classification group III (explained SUDI): cause of death

Cause of death	Number ascertained		Number interviewed with controls	
	n = 93	*%*	*n = 72*	*%*
Infections*	35	37.6	32	44.4
Accidental death	15	16.1	11	15.3
Non-accidental injury	21	22.6	9	12.5
Congenital abnormality	10	10.8	10	13.9
Intestinal obstruction	5	5.4	5	6.9
Metabolic disorder	4	4.3	4	5.6
Other†	3	3.2	1	1.4

* Includes meningitis, septicaemia, bronchopneumonia, gastro-enteritis and myocarditis

† Bronchopulmonary dysplasia, cardiac rhabdomyoma, cardiomyopathy

These figures do not represent the typical pattern of causation for infant mortality as a whole because they do not include deaths in the first week of life, expected deaths and SIDS.

Temporal factors

Age distribution

Figure 3.2 shows the distribution of explained SUDI deaths by four-week intervals of age. More deaths occurred in the first four weeks than in any later period, despite the fact that this period was a week shorter than the rest because deaths in the first week were excluded. After the first eight weeks, there was no obvious pattern to the frequency of deaths. This is in contrast with the characteristic distribution of SIDS deaths, which are uncommon in the first month of life, rise to a peak at 12 weeks and then decline steadily to almost zero by 11 months.

Figure 3.2   Age distribution of explained SUDI

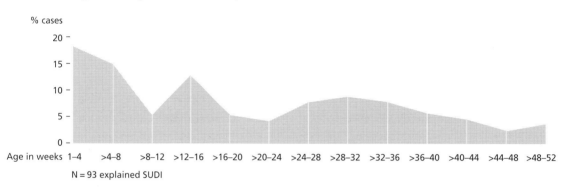

N = 93 explained SUDI

Incidence by season and days of the week

There was some seasonal variation in the incidence of explained deaths, with most (14 out of 93) occurring in December and fewest (4 out of 93) in April and August. There was no significant difference between the numbers of deaths occurring on different days of the week.

Factors relating to the infant

Amongst the explained SUDI, there was a higher proportion of boys than girls (61.1%) than amongst the controls (50.7%) but this was not statistically significant (OR = 1.57 [0.85–2.87]). The birth weight of infants who died was on average 281 g less than that of controls, and significantly more of the explained SUDI infants, 12 of 70 (17.1%) vs. 15 of 276 controls (5.4%) weighed less than 2,500 g at birth (OR = 3.28 [1.27–8.45]). Similarly, the gestational age of babies who died was on average five days less than that of controls, significantly more, 21 of 68 (30.9%) vs. 21 of 275 controls (7.6%), being born before 38 weeks (OR = 6.52 [2.66–15.99]). Fewer of the index babies were ever breast-fed 30 of 63 (47.6%) vs. 161 of 288 controls (55.9%), the difference not being significant (OR = 1.39 [0.72–2.66]).

Factors relating to the mother

The mean age of index mothers was 29 months less than that of controls, and significantly more (58.3% vs 40.8% controls) were aged under 27 years (OR = 2.09 [1.13–3.84]). Index mothers were more likely to have had at least three previous children, but were less likely to have the support of a partner. Significantly more index than control mothers smoked during pregnancy 30 of 61 (49.2%) vs. 81 of 288 (28.1%): OR = 3.54 [1.74–7.18]), and a dose-response effect was found whereby the association increased with the number of cigarettes smoked. In addition, according to parents' estimates index babies were exposed to a smoky atmosphere for longer periods each day than were control babies, with significantly more of the index babies (24 of 58 (41.4%) vs. 76 of 287 controls (26.5%) exposed for at least one hour (OR = 2.99 [1.44–6.21]).

Socio-economic factors

Index parents were more likely to be unemployed at the time of interview 32 of 67 (47.8%) vs. 44 of 288 controls (15.3%): OR = 5.56 [2.68–11.56]), and to be receiving Income Support 38 of 60 (63.3%) vs. 78 of 288 controls (27.1%): OR = 3.85 [1.96–7.56]). Figure 3.3 shows the occupational classification of index families and controls, using the highest present or previous occupation of either parent (I being the highest). Proportionately more of the index families were classified as socio-economic class (SEC) III manual, IV, V and unemployed compared to the controls, this difference was significant (OR = 2.11 [1.06–4.20]). Index parents were also more likely to have no basic educational qualification, to be living in accommodation that was rented and more crowded, and to have no access to a telephone.

Recent illness in the baby

The study questionnaire included a number of questions from the Cambridge 'Baby Check', a system devised to help doctors and carers assess the severity of illness in babies up to six months of age [3]. This system has a list of easily recognised symptoms and signs, each of which is scored, the sum of the scores giving a guide to the severity of the illness. A total score of less than eight indicates that the baby is generally well, while a score between eight and 12 suggests that the baby is unwell but not seriously ill, and the carers are advised to get advice and observe how the baby progresses. A score of more than 12 indicates that the baby is ill and needs a doctor, and if the score is over 19 the baby is seriously ill and needs a doctor straight away. Table 3.5 shows the number of index babies who had a score of more than 12 in the previous 24 hours before death as compared with controls before reference sleep.

Table 3.5 Health of infant in last 24 hours

Baby Check score	explained SUDI		Controls		OR (95% CI)
	n = 61	%	n = 288	%	
12 or less	34	55.7	280	97.2	1.00 (reference group)
>12 (required medical attention)	27	44.3	8	2.8	22.02 (6.86–70.94)

A striking finding was that, according to retrospective scoring by the Baby Check system, 44.3% of the index babies had been in need of medical attention in the previous 24 hours as compared with only 2.8% of controls, a difference that yielded a very high odds ratio. Of the 27 index babies with scores >12 (who needed medical attention), 2 of 27 (7.4%) had not been seen by any health professional in the week before they died, while 9 of 25 (36.0%) of those who had been seen were pronounced to have nothing wrong with them.

Summary of the findings of case-control study for 'explained SUDI' *

■   The highest proportion of deaths occurred in the first month of life.

---

* These findings have previously been published in detail in the Fifth Annual Report of CEDSI London: Maternal and Child Health Research Consortium, 1998. ISBN 0 9533536 0 5.

- The peak incidence of deaths was in December.

- The babies who died were of lower birth weight and shorter gestational age than the controls.

- The mothers of the infants who died were generally younger but started their families earlier than those of controls.

- The parents of the infants who died had lower educational attainments, were more commonly unemployed or in the less skilled occupation groups than those of controls.

- The families of infants who died were more likely to be in receipt of Income Support than were those of controls.

- Accommodation for index families was more likely to be rented and to be overcrowded than for controls.

- Babies who died more commonly had evidence of illness in the previous 24 hours than controls.

- Index mothers were more likely to have smoked in pregnancy and their infants were more likely to have been regularly exposed to a smoky atmosphere than for controls.

Figure 3.3 Occupational classification of explained SUDI families and age-matched controls

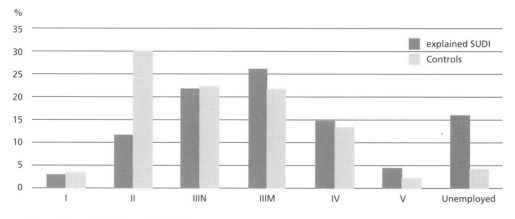

N = explained SUDI (67); controls (283)

EPIDEMIOLOGICAL FEATURES OF SIDS INFANTS*

Unless otherwise stated, this analysis uses the data from the 325 SIDS infants and their 1,300 matched controls.

Temporal factors

Age distribution

The median age of SIDS infants was 13 weeks (interquartile range: 7 weeks 6 days to 21 weeks 3 days). As previously noted, the median age of the control infants was 11 days greater, which is reflected in the slight shift of the age distribution amongst the controls towards the right (Figure 3.4).

---

* A comparison of epidemiological features of SIDS and explained SUDI infants has been published in full in *Pediatrics* (1999). See Appendix II for a full reference.

Figure 3.4 Age distribution of SIDS and control infants

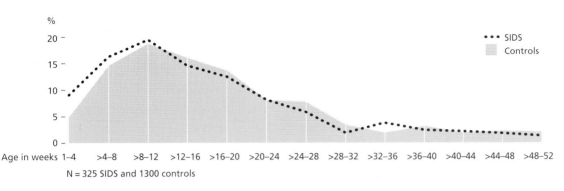

Age in weeks: 1–4 >4–8 >8–12 >12–16 >16–20 >20–24 >24–28 >28–32 >32–36 >36–40 >40–44 >44–48 >48–52

N = 325 SIDS and 1300 controls

Seasonality

The monthly fluctuation of deaths was small, ranging from 12.7% of deaths occurring in March to 4.9% in August (Figure 3.5). The distribution range by month of birth was even narrower, between 6.5% and 9.5% of births occurring in each month except December, in which 12.1% of the SIDS infants were born.

Figure 3.5 Seasonal occurrence of birth and deaths amongst SIDS infants

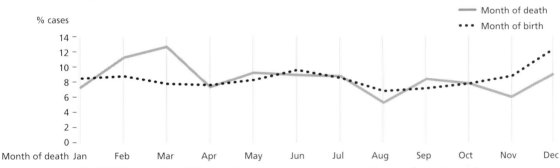

N = 306 SIDS (excluding 19 Trent deaths occurring during an incomplete year of ascertainment)

Day of death

A higher proportion of deaths occurred on Thursdays and Fridays, a smaller proportion on Tuesdays and Saturdays (Table 3.6). The distribution amongst the controls was not random, as most of these interviews were conducted between Monday and Friday. Comparing the distribution of day of death to a uniform distribution, there was significant (chi-squared test $p = 0.04$) variation in day of the week on which deaths occurred (Table 3.6).

Time death discovered

Of the 325 SIDS deaths, 55 (16.9%) occurred during daytime sleep. The 'reference' sleep of 93.6% of the control infants was matched to the index daytime or night-time sleep. Figure 3.6 compares the time the deaths were discovered with the times the control infants awoke from their reference sleep. The patterns are similar, 64.1% of the deaths were discovered, and 66.3% of the controls awoke, between 5.30 a.m. and 11.30 a.m. The time of discovery of the deaths was, on average, approximately one hour later than the times at which the controls awoke. This could suggest either that the sleeping patterns of the SIDS infants were different from the control infants (SIDS infants usually woke later) or that the deaths were discovered approximately one hour after the time SIDS infants usually awoke (or the parents usually awoke).

Table 3.6 Day of death

Day of death	n = 325	%
Monday	53	16.3
Tuesday	32	9.8
Wednesday	44	13.5
Thursday	56	17.2
Friday	59	18.2
Saturday	38	11.7
Sunday	43	13.2

Compared to a uniform distribution (i.e. equal proportions for each day) there was a significant departure (chi-squared test $p = 0.04$), but no one particular day when the number of deaths was significantly different than expected

Figure 3.6 Time death was discovered and control infants awoke

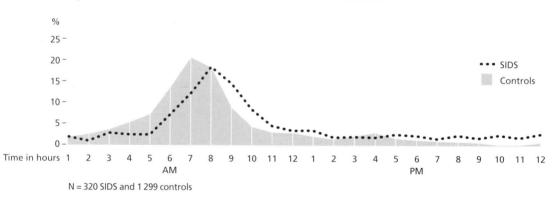

N = 320 SIDS and 1 299 controls

Time infants were put down to sleep

In the third year of the study, information was collected on the time infants were put down for the last or reference sleep (Figure 3.7). This suggests that the sleeping patterns of the two groups of families were different. Of the control infants, 50.9% were put down to sleep between the hours of 7.30pm and 11.30pm, compared with 27.4% of the SIDS infants. Conversely, 28.3% of the SIDS infants compared with 15.7% of the controls were put to bed between the hours of 12.30am and 4.30am.

Figure 3.7 Time infant was put down to sleep (third year only)

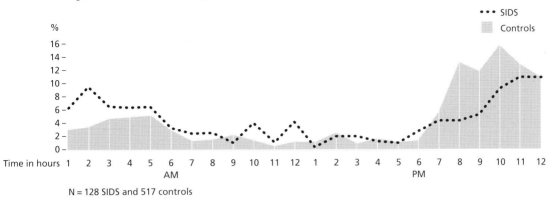

N = 128 SIDS and 517 controls

Interval from being put down to being discovered or waking

Data from the third year of the study (Figure 3.8) show the interval from when the infant was put down to the time the infant was discovered dead or awoke. There is a bi-modal distribution, with peaks at three hours and again at eight to nine hours. The median interval for index infants was 4.2 hours (interquartile range: 2.4–7.5 hours) compared to six hours for control infants (interquartile range: 2.9–9 hours). Using five to eight hours as a reference group, the risk associated with shorter intervals (zero to four hours) was not significant (OR = 1.31 [95% CI: 0.82–2.1]) but the protective effect of longer intervals (> eight hours) was significant (OR = 0.51 [95% CI: 0.29–0.91].

Figure 3.8 Interval from being put down to being found (third year only)

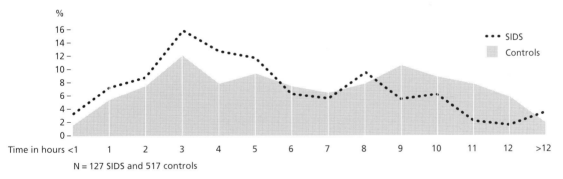

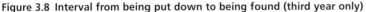

N = 127 SIDS and 517 controls

Infant factors

Gender

The proportion of boys was significantly higher amongst the SIDS infants than the controls (63.1% vs. 51.7%) (OR = 1.66 [95% CI: 1.26–2.18]).

Birth weight

The median birth weight for SIDS infants (3,053 g [interquartile range: 2,575–3,458 g]) was significantly lower than for the controls (3,399 g [interquartile range: 3,080–3,692 g]) (p < 0.0001). Figure 3.9 shows that a greater proportion of SIDS infants had birth weights below 3,250 g.

Figure 3.9 Birth weight

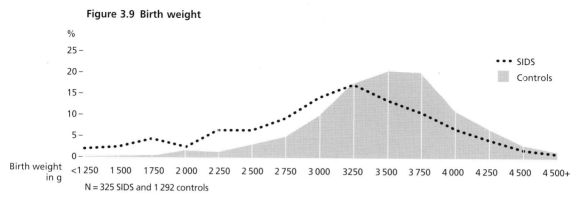

N = 325 SIDS and 1 292 controls

Gestation

For SIDS infants, the median gestation (38 weeks and 1 day [interquartile range: 36 weeks 4 days to 39 weeks 3 days]) was significantly shorter than for the controls (39 weeks 1 day [interquartile range: 38 weeks 1 day to 39 weeks 6 days]) ($p < 0.0001$) (Figure 3.10).

Figure 3.10 Gestation

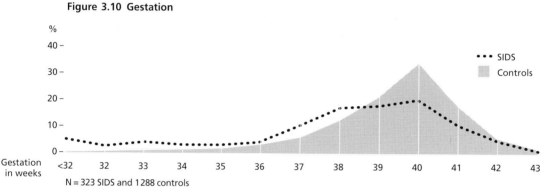

N = 323 SIDS and 1 288 controls

A similar proportion of infants (3.7% SIDS vs. 4.8% controls) were born at or beyond 42 weeks. Short gestation (below 40 weeks) was associated with an increased risk of SIDS (Table 3.7).

Table 3.7 Gestational age and the risk of SIDS

Gestation	SIDS		Controls		OR (95% CI)
	n = 323	%	n = 1 288	%	
40+ weeks	112	34.7	730	56.7	1.00 (reference group)
37–39 weeks	148	45.8	488	37.9	1.86 (1.38–2.51)
36 weeks or less	63	19.5	70	5.4	5.07 (3.29–7.80)

Centile at birth

Low birth weight and short gestation are partially correlated and boys are born, on average, heavier than girls, hence birth weight needs to be adjusted for these factors. To take account of these effects, z-scores (multiples of standard deviation from the normal mean) were calculated from sex-specific charts of birth weight and gestation [4] for SIDS and controls (Figure 3.11).

Figure 3.11 Centiles at birth (z-scores)

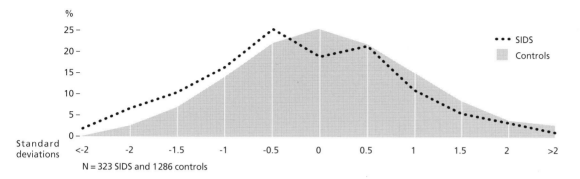

N = 323 SIDS and 1286 controls

A characteristic, symmetrical distribution, centred around zero, is seen for control infants, but for SIDS infants the distribution is shifted towards the left. The median z-score for SIDS cases was -0.3 standard deviations (interquartile range: -0.9 to +0.5 standard deviations) compared to zero for controls (interquartile range: -0.6 to +0.7 standard deviations). As a continuous variable adjusted for matching, the birth weight centile was significant ($p < 0.0001$). If the adjusted birth weight centile variable ($p < 0.0001$) and the variables for gestational age ($p < 0.0001$) and sex ($p = 0.01$) are put into a multiple logistical regression model, all three variables remain significant. Hence, the lower birth weight of the SIDS infants is not due solely to their shorter gestation.

Problems at delivery

Place of delivery

The vast majority of SIDS and control infants were born in hospital (97.2% vs. 98.3%), seven SIDS and 21 control infants were delivered at home but this difference was not statistically significant (OR = 1.35 [95% CI: 0.48–3.33]). A further two SIDS and one control infant were born on the way to hospital.

Apgar scores and resuscitation at delivery

Significantly more of the SIDS infants (25.4% vs. 19.8%) had an Apgar score of below eight at one minute (OR = 1.50 [95% CI: 1.08–2.08]). The proportional difference was greater, and statistically significant, for scores below eight at five minutes (5.1% vs. 2.1%) (OR = 2.54 [95% CI: 1.28–5.05]).

More SIDS infants than controls needed resuscitation at delivery (28.3% vs. 25.1%), but this difference was not significant (OR = 1.18 [95% CI: 0.89–1.57]). For infants who were resuscitated using either intubation (5.6% SIDS, 1.6% controls) or cardiopulmonary respiration (CPR) (2.2% SIDS, 0.3% controls) the difference was proportionally greater, and statistically significant (OR = 4.11 [95% CI: 2.13–7.92]).

Admission to special care baby unit

Eighty out of 323 (24.8%) of the SIDS infants, and 92 of 1,291 (7.1%) of the controls were admitted to a special care baby unit (SCBU) (OR = 4.25 [95% CI: 2.91–6.21]). Of these, 62.5% of the SIDS infants and 39.1% of controls were less than 37 weeks' gestation. If preterm infants are excluded, the risk associated with admission to SCBU halved but still remained statistically significant (OR = 2.26 [95% CI: 1.39–3.66]). Table 3.8 shows the most common reasons for admission for both the preterm and term infants (for some infants, more than one reason was stated, the percentages are quoted using the denominators of 323 SIDS infants and 1,291 controls).

Table 3.8 Common reasons for admission to special care baby unit

Reason for admission	SIDS (n = 80/323)				Controls (n = 92/1291)			
	Pre-term	Term	All	%	Pre-term	Term	All	%
Common reasons								
Agitated/jittery/irritable	0	0	0	0	0	6	6	0.5
Birth asphyxia	0	1	1	0.3	2	2	4	0.3
Breathing difficulties*	20	5	25	7.7	14	25	39	3.0
Congenital abnormality	0	4	4	1.2	0	0	0	0
Growth retardation	5	6	11	3.4	5	2	7	0.5
Infection†	6	2	8	2.5	3	7	10	0.8
Jaundice/phototherapy	2	0	2	0.6	1	4	5	0.4
Poor feeding‡	4	8	12	3.7	3	5	8	0.6
Problems with blood sugar levels§	1	6	7	2.2	6	8	14	1.1
Temperature: hypothermia/cold	3	3	6	1.9	3	6	9	0.7
Pyrexia/hot	0	2	2	0.6	0	1	1	0.1
Other	7	10	17	5.3	6	18	24	1.9

* Includes: respiratory distress, needing ventilator, grunting, apnoea, nasal flaring, pneumothorax

† Infections: suspected or proven

‡ Includes: infants given naso-gastric tube, iv fluids, nil by mouth

§ Includes: gestational diabetes, hyperglycaemia, hypoglycaemia

Neonatal problems and congenital anomalies

Table 3.9 lists the congenital anomalies noted in the neonatal period for SIDS and control infants (none of the infants had more than one minor or major congenital anomaly).

Table 3.9 Congenital anomalies

Type of anomaly	SIDS				Controls			
	Minor	Major	All		Minor	Major	All	
			n = 323	%			n = 1 290	%
None			298	92.3			1 224	94.9
Positional deformity	1	3	4	1.2	15	13	28	2.2
Of genito-urinary system	2	2	4	1.2	6	11	17	1.3
Of cardiovascular system	1	5	6	1.9	1	0	1	0.1
Other malformation	5 *	6 †	11	3.4	17 ‡	3 §	20	1.6

* Umbilical hernia, floppy pinna, extra digit, missing digit, ductal murmur

† Face dysmorphic, cleft palate, extra thumb, blepharophimosis, aplasia cutis, facial palsy

‡ Three with birthmark, four with skin tag, three with sacral dimple, extra digit, umbilical hernia, overlapping toes, abnormal toe, wide sutures, systolic murmur, micrognathia

§ Cleft palate, bifid thumb and polydactyly, sacral cleft

More SIDS infants had congenital anomalies compared to controls but this was not significant (OR = 1.56 [95% CI: 0.94–2.57]). However, significantly more SIDS infants (5.0% vs. 2.1%) had major malformations (OR = 2.46 [95% CI: 1.20–5.07]), a third of which were cardiovascular.

Table 3.10 lists the neonatal problems identified for SIDS and control infants. On the rare occassion that a particular infant had more than one neonatal problem, the more serious problem was chosen. Significantly more of the SIDS infants had neonatal problems (OR = 2.72 [95% CI: 1.93–3.83]) and significantly more of these problems were major (OR = 3.91 [95% CI: 2.28–6.72]). Amongst the SIDS infants, the most common problems were respiratory and those related to preterm delivery.

Table 3.10 Neonatal problems

Type of problem	SIDS				Controls			
	Minor	Major	All		Minor	Major	All	
			n = 322	%			n = 1 291	%
None			239	74.2			1 148	88.9
Preterm delivery problems	3	13	16	5.0	2	7	9	0.7
Intrapartum asphyxia	4	2	6	1.9	9	11	20	1.5
Treating congenital anomalies	1	1	2	0.6	6	2	8	0.6
Infection	1	2	3	0.9	7	6	13	1.0
Feeding problems	3	1	4	1.2	6	1	7	0.5
Jaundice	8	2	10	3.1	13	4	17	1.3
Respiratory problems	5	10	15	4.7	12	5	17	1.3
Metabolic problems	4	1	5	1.6	12	3	15	1.2
Other problems	20 *	2 †	22	6.8	35 *	2 ‡	37	2.9

* Includes: jittery infant, soft murmurs, misshapen head, infant cold, umbilical hernia, discharging eyes

† Includes: fetal alcohol syndrome, hypothermia

‡ Includes: blood sugar low at birth – renal scan, hypothermia

Treatments and procedures in the neonatal period

Several treatments/procedures undergone by infants in the neonatal period were more common amongst SIDS infants than controls, as shown in Table 3.11.

Maternal factors

Parity

This was based on the number of live births recorded in the mother's hospital records and checked against the number of children in the household. Where an obvious discrepancy occurred, the mother's response was taken. Index and control infants were included in the count. As a continuous variable, this factor was significant ($p < 0.0001$). Because of the limited number of categories, this variable is best represented as a multicategorical variable. Table 3.12 shows that, taking families with one child as the reference group, the risk of SIDS increased with increasing family size.

Table 3.11 Treatments and procedures in the neonatal period

	SIDS		Controls		OR (95% CI)
	n = 325	%	n = 1 300	%	
Intravenous fluids	48	14.8	42	3.2	5.08 (3.10–8.30)
Antibiotics	42	12.9	49	3.8	3.72 (2.29–6.04)
Added oxygen	26	8.0	20	1.5	5.29 (2.72–10.30)
IPPV/CPAP	26	8.0	13	1.0	7.90 (3.58–17.45)
Tube feeds	57	17.5	47	3.6	5.92 (3.68–9.50)
Phototherapy	35	10.8	34	2.6	4.02 (2.32–6.97)
Transfusions	7	2.2	7	0.5	4.66 (1.50–14.50)

The reference group are those of the 325 SIDS infants and 1,300 controls who did not receive the treatment or undergo the procedure listed

Table 3.12 Parity (including index or control infant)

Number of children	SIDS		Controls		OR (95% CI)
	n = 325	%	n = 1 300	%	
One child	90	27.7	558	42.9	1.00 (reference group)
Two children	94	28.9	454	34.9	} 1.78 (1.31–2.42)
Three children	85	26.2	188	14.5	
Four children	33	10.2	65	5.0	} 3.93 (2.52–6.12)
Five or more children	23	7.1	35	2.7	

Multiple births

Significantly more of the SIDS infants were twins or triplets compared to control infants (OR = 8.27 [95% CI: 3.41–20.05]). There were no instances of more than one death from one set of twins or triplets (see Table 3.13).

Table 3.13 Comparison of multiple births

	SIDS		Controls	
	n = 325	%	n = 1 300	%
Singleton	308	94.8	1 288	99.1
Twin	15	4.6	12	0.9
Triplet	2	0.6	0	0

Mother's past obstetric history

Previous stillbirths

Table 3.14 shows the number of previous stillbirths experienced by each mother. This question was asked in the interview and obtained from the records. If there was a discrepancy the mother's response was taken.

Table 3.14 Previous stillbirths

	SIDS		Controls	
	n = 325	%	n = 1 300	%
None	315	96.9	1 285	98.8
One	7	2.2	13	1.0
Two or more	3	0.9	2	0.2

A significant difference was found in the number of previous stillbirths between the SIDS and control mothers (OR = 2.82 [95% CI: 1.16–6.85]). Amongst the index mothers, there was one discrepancy (mother stated two stillbirths, whilst hospital records did not state any), amongst the control mothers there were five discrepancies (three mothers stated stillbirths [two stated two stillbirths, one stated one stillbirth] where none were recorded in the hospital records, and two control mothers did not mention a stillbirth but the hospital records stated one stillbirth). If we base the number of stillbirths on the hospital records rather than the information from the mothers, the difference between the two groups remains significant (OR = 3.13 [95% CI: 1.20–8.14]).

Previous termination of pregnancy

Whilst a higher proportion of the index (15.4%) than control mothers (12.5%) had undergone at least one previous termination of pregnancy, this did not achieve statistical significance (OR = 1.28 [95% CI: 0.89–1.82]).

Previous miscarriages

A higher proportion of the SIDS mothers (27.7%) than mothers of control infants (20.2%) had experienced at least one previous miscarriage (OR = 1.51 [95% CI: 1.11–2.04]).

Previous deaths of children in the family

No families had experienced previous deaths of children older than two years. No family had had more than one previous death except for one index and one control family in which both members of a pair of twins had died soon after birth. Table 3.15 shows the number and cause of all previous childhood deaths in index and control families. A previous infant had died in significantly more SIDS families than controls (4.0 % vs. 1.2%) (OR = 3.82 [95% CI: 1.58–9.22]). This previous death had been attributed to SIDS in five families of cases and two of controls (OR = 8.22 [95% CI: 1.56–43.24]). For one family (included in the above numbers), the two deaths attributed to SIDS were both included in this study, and for one family whose infant was included as a control during the first two years of the study, a subsequent baby died and was included as a SIDS infant in the third year. For two further families, in which a baby died during the first two years of the study and the death was attributed to SIDS, a subsequent infant death in the third year of the study was attributed to non-accidental injury.

Table 3.15 Previous infant deaths among siblings

Cause of death	SIDS (n = 323)		Controls (n = 1 288)	
	Deaths	%	Deaths	%
Infants < 1 year old				
SIDS	5	1.5	2	0.2
Extreme prematurity	2 *	0.6	9 *	0.7
Congenital abnormality	0	0	3	0.2
Infection	0	0	1	0.1
Ruptured hernia	1	0.3	0	0
Cerebral haemorrhage	1	0.3	0	0
Oligohydramnios	1	0.3	0	0
Infants 1–2 years old				
Congenital abnormality	1	0.3	0	0
Accidental	1	0.3	0	0
Infection	0	0	1	0.1
Hydrocephalus	1	0.3	0	0
Total	13	4.0	16	1.2

* Includes a set of twins to one family

Interpregnancy interval

Of the SIDS mothers, 239 (73.5%) had had a previous live birth, stillbirth, miscarriage or termination compared to 830 (63.8%) control mothers. For these mothers, the interval from the end of the last pregnancy to the last menstrual period prior to this birth is shown in Figure 3.12.

Figure 3.12 Interpregnancy interval

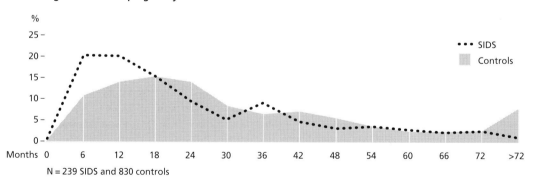

N = 239 SIDS and 830 controls

The interpregnancy interval was shorter for SIDS mothers (median = 16 months [interquartile range: 7–32 months]) than for control mothers (median = 23 months [interquartile range: 12–41 months]). This difference was significant both as a continuous variable ($p = 0.0002$) and as a dichotomous variable using seven months or more as the reference group (including first-time mothers) (OR = 2.33 [95% CI: 1.53–3.56]).

Immediate obstetric history

Antenatal booking

The number of weeks after the last menstrual period that obstetric/midwifery care was booked was ascertained from the medical records. The median number of weeks to booking for SIDS mothers was 13 weeks (interquartile range 10–17 weeks) compared to 11 weeks for control mothers (interquartile range 8–14 weeks). Three SIDS mothers and two controls did not book for obstetric or midwifery care. Taking booking within the first trimester as the reference group, later booking was significantly associated with an increased risk of SIDS, as shown in Table 3.16.

Table 3.16 Timing of initial booking for obstetric care

	SIDS		Controls		OR (95% CI)
	n = 309	%	n = 1 268	%	
First trimester	174	56.3	937	73.9	1.00 (reference group)
Second trimester	118	38.2	309	24.4	2.47 (1.78–3.43)
Third trimester*	17	5.5	22	1.7	5.40 (2.55–11.47)

* Including those mothers who did not book obstetric care

This was not the first birth for proportionately more of the SIDS mothers. If parity is added to the above variable, the time of booking medical care remains significant both for the second trimester (OR = 2.24 [95% CI: 1.60–3.14]) and the third trimester (OR = 4.82 [95% CI: 2.21–10.50]).

Pregnancy problems

Whilst anaemia, high blood pressure and urinary tract infections during pregnancy were all slightly more common amongst mothers of SIDS infants than controls, these differences were not statistically significant.

Labour and delivery

There was no difference in the incidence of spontaneous rupture of membranes, induction of labour or of augmentation of labour between mothers of SIDS and control infants. There was no significant difference between SIDS and controls in the place of birth (i.e. home, general practitioner unit, consultant unit), but more SIDS infants (13.7%) than controls (8.3%) were delivered by caesarean section (OR = 1.85 [95% CI: 1.22–2.81]).

Family factors

Infant adopted or fostered

Of the SIDS infants, six (1.8%) were adopted or fostered compared to eight control infants (0.6%). This factor was not significant (OR = 2.96 [95% CI: 0.88–9.96]).

Parental age

Maternal age

The median age of SIDS mothers was 23 years and 4 months (interquartile range: 19 years 11 months to 28 years 3 months) compared to 26 years and 11 months for control mothers (interquartile range: 23 years to 30 years 5 months), a difference of 3.5 years (Figure 3.13). The difference in maternal age, as a continuous variable, was highly significant ($p < 0.0001$).

Figure 3.13 Maternal age at delivery

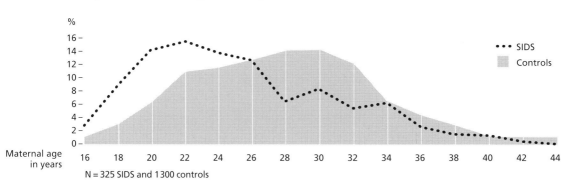

N = 325 SIDS and 1300 controls

Paternal age

The median age of partners of SIDS mothers was 27 years and 4 months (interquartile range: 23 years 2 months to 30 years 11 months) compared to 29 years for partners of control mothers (interquartile range: 25 years 5 months to 33 years 2 months). This difference is less significant than for maternal age ($p = 0.003$).

Parental age difference

Although it is clear that the index parents were younger, the above analysis does not indicate the age difference between parents. This was greater for index than control families, particularly for younger mothers, but, as a continuous variable, just failed to reach significance ($p = 0.052$).

Racial/ethnic group

Mother's ethnic group

Table 3.17 shows the ethnicity of index and control mothers. The vast majority of index and control mothers were white, and no significant ethnic differences were found.

Father's ethnic group

As for the mothers, the great majority of index fathers (88.4%) and control fathers were white (92.4%). There were no significant differences in ethnicity between SIDS and control fathers.

Mother's country of birth

More index than control mothers were born outside the UK (6.5% vs. 4.5%), but this difference was not significant (OR = 1.47 [0.85–2.52]).

Table 3.17 Mother's ethnic group

	SIDS		Controls	
	n = 324	%	n = 1 299	%
White	299	92.3	1 217	93.7
Black (Caribbean)	6	1.9	15	1.2
Black (African)	1	0.3	2	0.2
Black (other)	0	0	3	0.2
Indian	1	0.3	17	1.3
Pakistani	9	2.8	34	2.6
Bangladeshi	1	0.3	4	0.3
Chinese/Japanese	0	0	1	0.1
Mixed race	7	2.2	6	0.5

Father's country of birth

More of the index than control fathers were born outside the UK (7.2% vs. 5.9%), but this difference was not significant (OR = 1.43 [95% CI: 0.85–2.40]).

Marital status

Supported mothers were defined as those who had a partner, whether or not they were married or living together. Unsupported mothers included those who were separated, divorced or without a current partner; none of the mothers had been widowed. Data were collected on marital status at the time of conception, time of delivery and the time of interview. The details are given in Table 3.18.

Table 3.18 Marital status of mothers

Marital status at:		SIDS		Controls		OR (95% CI)
		n = 325	%	n = 1 300	%	
Conception	Supported	289	88.9	1 257	96.7	1.00 (reference group)
	Unsupported	36	11.1	43	3.3	4.17 (2.40–7.25)
Delivery	Supported	283	87.1	1 237	95.2	1.00 (reference group)
	Unsupported	42	12.9	63	4.8	3.21 (1.99–5.19)
Interview	Supported	280	86.2	1 231	94.7	1.00 (reference group)
	Unsupported	45	13.8	69	5.3	3.00 (1.89–4.77)

The proportion of unsupported mothers rose in both groups over time. The difference between the two groups also narrowed, although the difference remained significant for each time period.

Support from relatives and friends

The mother was asked if there was any support other than a partner she could turn to if she was worried about the baby for any reason. Three potential sources of support were identified: grandparents, other family and friends. The majority of mothers received support from all three sources, particularly grandparents, with no identifiable differences between the mothers of SIDS and control infants.

Access to health professionals and emergency services

Use of telephone in emergencies

The parents were asked whether there was a working telephone in the home from which outgoing calls could be made. Three times as many index as control families (41.7% vs. 13.9%) did not have a telephone in the home (OR = 4.97 [95% CI: 3.58–6.90]). If there was no telephone, most index and control families responded that there was a pay phone in the building or nearby in the street, or possible use of a neighbour's phone. However, of the index families, 4.4% had no access to a telephone within five minutes of travelling time, compared to 1.3% of the controls. This difference was significant (OR = 5.17 [95% CI: 2.09–12.80]).

Use of own transport

The parents were asked whether they had use of any type of motorised private transport. Significantly more of the index families (52.3%) than controls (22.9%) did not have their own transport (OR = 4.94 [95% CI: 3.59–6.80]). Nearly three-quarters (74.0%) of the index mothers had no transport of their own, could not drive, or had no access to their partner's transport compared to 43.5% of the control mothers (OR = 4.86 [95% CI: 3.48–6.77]).

Socio-economic factors

Family income and receipt of Income Support

Table 3.19 details the weekly income that came into the household, and whether the family was in receipt of Income Support, a means-tested benefit provided by the government for parents who are unemployed or on low income. In order to take account of the discrepancy between the marital status of SIDS and control mothers (as noted above), an additional analysis, in which we have controlled for whether the mother was supported by a partner at the time of interview, has been included in this table.

Only 12 of the SIDS families (3.7%) and 16 of the control families (1.2%) did not provide information on weekly income. The risk of SIDS was higher the lower the family income. Twice as many SIDS as control families received Income Support. Both findings remained statistically significant when controlled for whether the mother was supported by a partner. In the third year of the study, the mothers were asked whether the estimate of weekly income included the partner's contribution. Of the SIDS mothers, 24% did not include a contribution from the partner compared to 15.4% of the controls. Some of these mothers were single, for others their partners did not live in the same household, and for others the partner was unemployed and had little income to contribute. Of those mothers living with an employed partner, 1.5% of both SIDS and control mothers did not include any contribution from the partner.

Table 3.19 Weekly family income and receipt of income support

	SIDS		Controls		OR (95% CI)	OR (95% CI)*
Weekly income	n = 313	%	n = 1 284	%		
£200 +	76	24.3	663	51.6	1.00 (reference group)	1.00 (reference group)
£100 – < £200	102	32.6	363	28.3	2.82 (1.95–4.08)	2.73 (1.88–3.95)
£60 – < £100	97	31.0	219	17.1	4.57 (3.06–6.82)	4.22 (2.78–6.40)
< £60	38	12.1	39	3.0	9.56 (5.24–17.43)	8.61 (4.63–16.03)
Receipt of income support	n = 319	%	n = 1 295	%		
No	113	35.4	914	70.6	1.00 (reference group)	1.00 (reference group)
Yes	206	64.6	381	29.4	5.76 (4.15–7.99)	5.37 (3.83–7.52)

* Adjusted for whether the mother was supported by a partner at time of interview

Parental employment

Occupational classification

Social class coding is taken from the Office of Population Censuses and Surveys' *Standard Occupational Classification* (HMSO, 1990).

The categories are as follows:

  I Professional occupations

  II Managerial and technical occupations

  III Skilled occupations: (N) non-manual; (M) manual

  IV Partly skilled occupations

  V Unskilled occupations

Armed forces personnel, students and those unemployed are included as 'unclassifiable' within this system.

Until recently, the classification was based on the occupation of the 'head of the household', usually the male. Given the shifting trend of higher female employment status in the household, it was no longer appropriate to assume the male has the 'better' occupation. Classification in this study was based on the employment status of both partners, and the 'head of the household' was the one with the higher social class by employment status. The unemployed are less easily classified because they are not an homogeneous group; unemployed professionals and unemployed unskilled workers differ. This problem was overcome by classifying on the basis of their previous employment if both parents were currently unemployed. If the partner was not part of the household, the mother was treated as the single occupant of the household. Figure 3.14 compares the occupational classification of index and control households, using the higher classification of either parent (I being the highest), and their previous occupation if currently unemployed.

Figure 3.14 Occupational classification (including previous occupation)

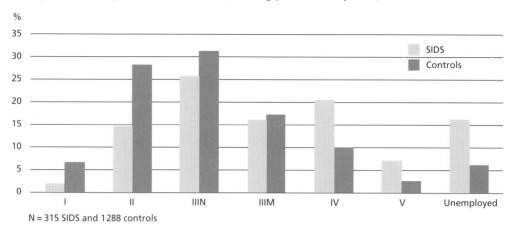

N = 315 SIDS and 1 288 controls

More control families were classified as social class I, II, IIIN and IIIM, whilst more SIDS families were classified as IV, V or unemployed. Even when previous employment was used, 16.2% of SIDS parents had never been employed, compared to 5.7% of control parents.

Of those not included in this figure, seven SIDS (2.2%) and eight control household occupations (0.6%) were classified as students. As two of the students were postgraduates and the rest had not exceeded GCSE status, one could reclassify them as social class II and unemployed, respectively. As a continuous variable, occupational classification is highly significant ($p < 0.0001$). Table 3.20 shows the social classification (including the student reclassification) as a multicategorical variable.

Table 3.20 Occupational classification

Social class	SIDS n = 322	%	Controls n = 1 296	%	OR [95% CI]
I and II	50	15.5	443	34.2	1.0 (reference group)
IIIN	80	24.8	402	31.0	1.76 (1.19–2.62)
IIIM, IV	113	35.1	344	26.5	2.91 (2.00–4.25)
V, Unemployed	79	24.5	107	8.3	6.54 (4.25–10.10)

Unemployment

Table 3.21 shows the number and proportion of unemployed parents in index and control families, divided into those in which the mother had or did not have a partner.

For mothers with a partner, nearly three times more SIDS than control parents were both unemployed. For those without a partner, 75.4% of control mothers and 95.5% SIDS mothers were unemployed. The proportion of SIDS and control households with no waged income (48.6% SIDS vs. 18.1% controls) were significantly different (OR = 4.59 [95% CI: 3.37–6.27]). The length of unemployment was similar in each group: 24 months for SIDS mothers (interquartile range 11–47 months), 23 months for control mothers (interquartile range 8–40 months), 11 months for SIDS partners (interquartile range 4–24 months) and 12 months for control partners (interquartile range 5–30 months).

Parental education

The level of education achieved by each parent is summarised in Table 3.22.

SIDS mothers and, to a slightly lesser extent their partners, had lower academic achievements than controls. Considering the highest qualification of either parent, the difference between the two groups is highly significant as a continuous variable ($p < 0.0001$). As a multi-categorical variable using attainment to 'A' level (or equivalent) or higher as the reference group, the risk associated with attainment to GCSE (OR = 1.13 [95% CI: 1.03–1.25]) and below GCSE (OR = 3.51 [95% CI: 2.39–5.15]) was significant.

Table 3.21 Unemployment

	SIDS	%	Controls	%	OR (95% CI)
Mothers with partners	*n = 279**	%	*n = 1 226[†]*	%	
Both employed	42	15.1	465	37.9	1.00 (reference group)
Only mother employed	9	3.2	41	3.3	2.43 (0.97–5.52)
Only partner employed	113	40.5	538	43.9	2.33 (1.57–3.45)
Both unemployed	115	41.2	182	14.8	7.00 (4.64–10.57)
Mothers without partners	*n = 44[‡]*	%	*n = 69*	%	
Employed	2	4.5	17	24.6	1.00 (reference group)
Unemployed	42	95.5	52	75.4	6.87 (1.47–63.75)

* One SIDS case missing

[†] Five controls missing

[‡] One SIDS case missing

Table 3.22 Parental education

Qualification or equivalent	Mother		Partner		Parents*	
	n = 316	n = 1 293	n = 262	n = 1 149	n = 317	n = 1 294
	SIDS %	controls %	SIDS %	controls %	SIDS %	controls %
Degree	2.8	7.3	4.6	11.4	4.4	12.9
Higher education	2.5	8.5	4.2	7.5	5.4	9.4
A level	5.4	8.8	7.6	10.0	8.2	12.9
GCSE level	25.0	33.0	23.3	27.7	30.3	35.4
Below GCSE level	23.4	23.4	24.4	23.6	25.6	18.3
None	40.8	18.9	35.9	19.8	26.2	11.1

* Highest qualification of either mother or partner

Type of accommodation

Type of housing

SIDS and control families lived in a wide range of housing types, with no significant differences between the groups other than more control than SIDS families were living in detached houses (11.8% vs. 6.2%, respectively), and more SIDS families were living in mobile homes, bed and breakfast or hostel accommodation (3.3% vs. no controls).

Tenure of housing

The types of housing tenure varied, but significantly more control (60.6%) than SIDS (25.3%) families owned their home or had a mortgage (OR = 5.07 [95% CI: 3.67–7.01]).

Council tax band

At the time of this study the Council 'tax band' house-rating system was relatively new and many index (39.7%) and control parents (25.1%) did not know their category. However, significantly more control (12.5%) than index families (5.6%) lived in higher-rated accommodation (bands D, E, F and G) (OR = 2.35 [95% CI: 1.08–5.10]).

Problems with accommodation

Condition of house

Families were asked about the presence and severity of damp, mould and water leaks in their home. All were more common and more severe in the homes of SIDS families. Comparing families whose homes had no problem or no serious problem with those whose homes had fairly or very serious problems, the risk of SIDS was higher in homes with damp (OR = 2.20 [95% CI: 1.54–3.12], mould (OR = 3.41 [95% CI: 2.21–5.25] and water leaks (OR = 2.77 [95% CI: 1.70–4.50]). Clearly, these problems are related. Table 3.23 combines the data for these three problems and also shows the proportion of households in which these problems specifically affected the infant's place of sleep.

In the presence of any of the problems of damp, mould or water leaking, the risk of SIDS increased with the seriousness of the reported problem, regardless of whether or not the problem was specifically reported as affecting the infant's place of sleep.

Overcrowding

The median number of rooms, excluding the bathroom, toilet if separate, hallways and kitchen (if not used as a dining room) in the index household was four (interquartile range: three to five rooms), whilst the median number in the control household was five (interquartile range: four to five rooms). Proportionally more of the SIDS families (26.9%) than controls (17.1%) had three rooms or fewer (OR = 1.78 [95% CI: 1.32–2.39]).

The median number of people (including all adults, children and infants) living in all households was four (interquartile range: three to five people). Because a greater proportion of index mothers were single, a larger proportion of index households had just two people in the household (index mother and baby). Conversely, because the index mothers' parity was higher, a larger proportion of index households also had larger families. Using three or four people per household as a reference group, significantly more index households had just two people (OR = 3.13 [95% CI: 1.58–6.15]) and also five people or more (OR = 2.19 [95% CI: 1.68–2.86]).

Table 3.23 Damp, mould and water leaks anywhere in the home and specifically affecting the infant's place of sleep

	SIDS		Controls		OR (95% CI)
	n = 320	%	n = 1 297	%	
Anywhere in the home					
None	176	55.0	830	64.0	1.00 (reference group)
Not serious	73	22.8	317	24.4	1.09 (0.79–1.48)
Fairly serious	48	15.0	124	9.6	1.83 (1.24–2.69)
Very serious	23	7.2	26	2.0	4.17 (2.24–7.77)
Affecting the infant's place of sleep					
None	270	84.4	1 197	92.3	1.00 (reference group)
Not serious	12	3.8	44	3.4	1.21 [0.60 to 2.41]
Fairly serious	26	8.1	44	3.4	2.62 [1.54 to 4.45]
Very serious	12	3.8	12	0.9	4.43 [1.80 to 10.90]

Dividing the number of people in the household by the number of rooms, a measure of overcrowding can be derived (e.g. if three people shared six rooms, the score would be 0.5). The median number of people per room for the index families was 0.94 (interquartile range: 0.77–1.30) and for control families it was 0.80 (interquartile range: 0.67–0.98 persons). As a continuous variable, the difference was highly significant ($p < 0.0001$). Twice as many index families as controls (40.3% vs. 21.9%) lived in accommodation where there was less than one room available for each member of the household (OR = 2.43 [95% CI: 1.81–3.27]).

Pets

A similar proportion of index (50.2%) and control households (52.6%) had at least one pet (OR = 0.91 [95% CI: 0.70–1.17]). Slightly more index families owned dogs (27% vs. 22%), and slightly more control families owned cats (24% vs. 20%), but neither difference was statistically significant. Two or more dogs were owned by 8% of SIDS families, compared to 5% of control families, which was just statistically significant (OR = 1.73 [95% CI: 1.03–2.87]).

UNIVARIATE ANALYSIS OF POTENTIALLY MODIFIABLE RISK FACTORS

Interpretation of the univariate results

Many of the factors presented in this and the previous section are intertwined and form complex relationships dependent on one another. To understand these relationships, these factors need to be looked at together in a multivariate analysis (presented later). Detailed univariate statistics are presented here to demonstrate the prevalence of individual factors within SIDS and control families.

It is important to emphasise that neither univariate analysis in isolation nor multivariate analysis without careful interpretation and confirmation from similar studies can give the 'full picture' of which factors contribute significantly to the risk of SIDS.

Sleeping position*

Usual sleeping position

The usual position in which SIDS and control infants were put down to sleep for both night and day sleeps is shown in Table 3.24.

Table 3.24 Usual sleeping position

Put down for:	SIDS		Controls		OR (95% CI)
Night sleeps	n = 321	%	n = 1 298	%	
Back	156	48.6	873	67.3	1.00 (reference group)
Side	128	39.9	389	30.0	1.76 (1.31–2.36)
Front	37	11.5	36	2.8	7.85 (4.41–13.95)
Day sleeps	n = 317	%	n = 1 283	%	
Back	176	55.5	946	73.7	1.00 (reference group)
Side	108	34.1	301	23.5	1.82 (1.34–2.47)
Front	33	10.4	36	2.8	7.71 (4.21–14.11)

The practice for day and night sleeps was similar. The prone position was the least used but carried the greatest risk. Side-sleeping position carried a significantly increased risk when compared with supine.

Table 3.25 contains data for the 128 SIDS infants (39.9%) and the 389 controls (30%) usually put down on their side for night sleeps, and examines whether the infant was put down on the right or the left side, and whether the lower arm was extended to help prevent the infant rolling into the prone

---

* Data from the first two years has been published in full in the *British Medical Journal* (1996). See Appendix II for a full reference.

position. The reference group were those infants who usually slept in the supine position at night. The percentages are based on all SIDS or control infants, regardless of sleep position.

The risk associated with left or right side was similar and statistically significant for both. The risk associated with the side position when the infant's lower arm was not extended was slightly higher than when the arm was extended.

Table 3.25 The effects of usually being put down on the right or the left side, and of having the lower arm extended when put down on the side for night sleeps

Usual night sleep	SIDS		Controls		OR (95% CI) *
	n = 321	%	n = 1 298	%	
Left side	45	14.0	148	11.4	1.71 (1.15–2.52)
Right side	38	11.8	129	9.9	1.65 (1.08–2.50)
Side (varied)†	45	14.0	112	8.6	2.25 (1.50–3.36)
	n = 321	%	n = 1 298	%	
Without arm extended	41	12.8	103	7.9	2.24 (1.47–3.40)
With arm extended	42	13.1	174	13.4	1.36 (0.91–2.01)
Side (varied)‡	45	14.0	112	8.6	2.25 (1.50–3.36)

* The reference group were those infants put down supine

† Infants sometimes put down on the right side and sometimes on the left

‡ Infants sometimes have lower arm extended and sometimes not when put down on their side

Change in sleeping position for usual sleeps

Overall, the SIDS infants tended to change their position during sleep less often than the controls, but this difference was not significant. Some infants were put down in one position and commonly found in another, particular position. Others moved into different positions, dependent on infant age. No single change in position was significantly different between SIDS and control infants.

Sleeping position for the last/reference sleep

The positions in which the SIDS infants and the controls were put down to sleep and found after the last or reference sleep are shown in Table 3.26.

Findings for the last/reference sleep correspond to the usual practice in that the prone position was the least common but carried the greatest risk. More SIDS and control infants were found prone than were put down in this position; this difference was much greater for the SIDS infants. Again, the side-sleeping position was associated with a significantly increased risk compared to the supine position.

Table 3.26 Sleeping position for the last/reference sleep

Position put down	SIDS		Controls		OR (95% CI)
	n = 317	%	n = 1 295	%	
Back	141	44.5	895	69.1	1.00 (reference group)
Side	129	40.7	361	27.9	2.19 (1.62–2.95)
Front	47	14.8	39	3.0	10.23 (5.92–17.68)
Position found	n = 306	%	n = 1 248	%	
Back	116	37.9	1 037	83.1	1.00 (reference group)
Side	76	24.8	134	10.7	4.74 (3.14–7.17)
Front	114	37.3	77	6.2	21.49 (12.98–35.58)

Table 3.27 contains data for the 129 SIDS infants (40.7%) and the 361 controls (27.9%) put down on their side for the last/reference sleep. The reference group was those infants who were put down in the supine position for this sleep. The percentages are based upon all SIDS or control infants regardless of sleep position.

Table 3.27 The effects of being put down on the right or the left side, and of having the lower arm extended for the last/reference sleeps

	SIDS		Controls		OR (95% CI) *
	n = 317	%	n = 1 295	%	
Left side	54	17.0	164	12.7	2.09 (1.44–3.02)
Right side	49	15.5	157	12.1	1.98 (1.35–2.90)
Side (unspecified)†	26	8.2	40	3.1	4.13 (2.36–7.19)
	n = 317	%	n = 1 295	%	
Without arm extended	47	14.8	116	9.0	2.57 (1.72–3.83)
With arm extended	56	17.7	205	15.8	1.73 (1.21–2.48)
Side (unspecified)†	26	8.2	40	3.1	4.13 (2.36–7.19)

* The reference group is those infants put down supine

† Parents indicated infant was put down on their side but did not specify whether this was the right or left side or whether the lower arm was extended

Findings for the last/reference sleep again correspond to the usual practice in that the risk was similar for those infants put down on their left or right side, and there was an increased risk for those infants who did not have their lower arm extended.

Change in sleeping position for the last/reference sleep

A similar proportion of index and control infants (27.5%, 24.3%, respectively) changed position during the last/reference sleep, and the ages of those who did were similar for both groups (median 97 and 99 days, respectively). However, infants put down on their sides and found in a different position were younger for both SIDS and controls (median 82 and 94 days, respectively) than those who moved from supine or prone positions (median 129 and 189 days, respectively). This suggests that a change from the side position may reflect the instability of the younger infants, whilst movement from a prone or supine position occurs mainly in older infants who have learned to roll over. The presumed stability of infants with their lower arm extended had little effect, as more than half of the infants who were put down on their side and moved to the supine or prone position had the lower arm extended.

The risk associated with changes in position is shown in Table 3.28.

Table 3.28 Risk associated with change in sleeping position

Position	SIDS		Controls		OR (95% CI)*	OR (95% CI)†
	n = 305	%	n = 1 246	%		
Put down and found on back	105	34.4	802	64.4	1.00 (reference group)	1.00 (reference group)
Moved to back	11	3.6	234	18.8	0.36 (0.18, 0.70)	
Put down and found on side	71	23.3	111	8.9	4.89 (3.35, 7.12)	5.71 (3.95, 8.27)
Moved to side	5	1.6	23	1.8	1.66 (0.48, 4.59)	1.94 (0.57, 5.35)
Put down and found on front	45	14.8	30	2.4	11.46 (6.72, 19.58)	13.40 (7.90, 22.78)
Moved to front	68	22.3	46	3.7	11.29 (7.22, 17.69)	13.20 (8.49, 20.55)

* Using as the reference group those infants put down and found on their backs

† Using as the reference group all those infants found on their backs

Significantly more control than SIDS infants rolled from the side to the back. There was a significant risk associated with being put down and remaining on the side. The risk associated with the prone position was similar for infants who moved into this position as for those who were put down into this position.

Summary of risks of sleeping position

The risk associated with the prone sleeping position was statistically significant, both for the infant's usual position during night or day sleeps, and for the last/reference sleep. A significant risk was associated with the lateral sleeping position, both for usual and for the last/reference sleep, regardless of whether infants were put down on the right or left sides, although the risk was reduced if the lower arm was extended. The move from side to prone position was more common amongst SIDS, and side to supine more common for control infants. Infants who moved from the side position to either the prone or supine position were generally younger than those who moved from the prone or supine positions. The risk associated with the prone position was similar, regardless of whether infants were placed in that position or moved to it from another position.

Thermal environment and arrangement of bedding*

Maternal anxiety over infant's thermal environment

Some mothers worry about their baby getting too cold, others worry about the baby getting too hot. The mothers were asked which they worried about most (Table 3.29).

Table 3.29 Maternal anxiety over infant's thermal environment

Mother worried about:	SIDS		Controls		OR (95% CI)*	OR (95% CI)†
	n = 317	%	n = 1 298	%		
Neither	61	19.2	226	17.4	1.00 (reference group)	1.00 (reference group)
Too hot or cold	87	27.4	303	23.3	1.06 (0.72–1.57)	
Too cold	88	27.8	205	15.8	1.59 (1.07–2.36)	1.51 (1.07–2.14)
Too hot	81	25.6	564	43.5	0.53 (0.36–0.78)	0.51 (0.36–0.71)

* Using as the reference group mothers who did not worry about their baby becoming either too hot or too cold

† Using as the reference group mothers who worried both about their baby becoming too hot and too cold, together with those who worried about neither

Significantly more control than index mothers worried about their baby getting too hot, suggesting a protective effect, whilst significantly more of the index mothers worried about their baby becoming too cold.

Tog values of bedding and clothing

Information was collected on the type, arrangement and number of layers of bedding and clothing, from which the total thermal resistance was calculated in togs (the tog value of a fabric is defined as 10 times the temperature difference in degrees Celsius between its two faces when the heat flow is equal to 1 Watt/square metre). Thus the higher the tog value of the bedding and clothing the more effective the insulation provided, i.e. the more warmly wrapped the baby will be. It is important to note that, whilst bedding with a high tog value is regarded as 'heavy' wrapping, there is no good relationship between the *weight* of bedding and its insulating properties. For example, duvets filled with down or hollow fibres are very light in weight, but very effective insulators, with correspondingly high tog values. Whilst the tog values for adult duvets are usually given on the manufacturer's label, this is less commonly the case for infant quilts or duvets. The tog values for the various items of bedding used were obtained from tables of materials and manufacturers supplied by the Shirley Institute in Manchester [1,5]. The effective thermal insulation of the bedding was calculated, taking into account the proportion of the baby's surface area which was covered by the bedding and clothing. Thus, a cot quilt of thermal insulation 5 tog which covered 80% of the baby would be considered as having an effective thermal resistance of 4 tog [5,6]. Whilst this approach does take some account of the proportion of the baby's surface covered by differing arrangements of bedding, it underestimates the additional effect of head covering [1,5,6,34].

---

* Data from the first two years has been published in full in the British Medical Journal (1996). See Appendix II for a full reference.

Thermal resistance was calculated for all clothing except the nappy, the tog value of which varies substantially, dependant upon the level of saturation.

The median tog values for the usual night and day sleeps, and when put down and found for the last/reference sleep, are shown in Table 3.30.

Table 3.30 Tog values of bedding and clothing for usual sleep and last/reference sleep

	SIDS	Controls	Significance
Usual night sleeps	**n = 321**	**n = 1 299**	
Median	5.25	4.70	p < 0.0001*
Interquartile range	2.90–8.05	2.72–6.56	
Proportion ≥ 10 tog	52 (16.2%)	108 (8.3%)	OR = 2.13 [1.47 to 3.09]†
Usual day sleeps	**n = 321**	**n = 1 298**	
Median	2.96	1.93	p < 0.0001*
Interquartile range	1.21–4.92	0.76–3.63	
Proportion ≥ 10 tog	21 (6.5%)	31 (2.4%)	OR = 2.86 [1.56 to 5.22]†
Put down last sleep	**n = 320**	**n = 1 299**	
Median	5.02	4.19	p < 0.0001*
Interquartile range	2.31–8.11	2.24–6.13	
Proportion ≥ 10 tog	56 (17.5%)	101 (7.8%)	OR = 2.54 [1.76 to 3.67]†
Found last sleep	**n = 319**	**n = 1 299**	
Median	3.73	2.71	p < 0.0001*
Interquartile range	1.33–7.66	0.73–5.38	
Proportion ≥ 10 tog	48 (15.0%)	68 (5.2%)	OR = 3.21 [2.13 to 4.38]†

* As a continuous variable

† As a dichotomous variable (reference group being those infants covered in < 10 tog)

For both the usual sleep and last/reference sleep, the SIDS infants were wrapped significantly more warmly than the control infants. The difference in the distribution of tog values remained significant when adjusted for socio-economic status. Notably twice as many SIDS infants put down for the last/reference sleep were covered by 10 tog or more of clothing or bedding, and three times as many were found this way compared to the control infants.

Using a sleeping bag or baby nest

More SIDS infants used a sleeping bag or baby nest for the usual sleep, both at night (OR = 3.18 [95% CI: 1.64–6.17]) and in the day (OR = 1.43 [95% CI: 0.82–2.50]). A similar difference (6.2% SIDS vs 1.8% controls) was found for the last/reference sleep (OR = 2.69 [95% CI: 1.34–5.34]).

Wearing a hat

Very few infants usually wore hats for their night sleeps, but significantly more of the SIDS (2.8%) than control infants (0.3%) did so (OR = 9.13 [95% CI: 2.22–37.60]). Usually wearing a hat for daytime sleeps was much more common, and similar between the two groups (9.3% SIDS vs. 9.2% controls). For the last/reference sleep, (including both day and night sleeps), significantly more of the SIDS (4.7%) than the control infants (1.8%) wore hats (OR = 3.12 [95% CI: 1.39–7.01]).

Use of an electric blanket

Very few of the babies were given an electric blanket either usually or at the time of the last sleep. At the time of the last/reference sleep, two SIDS infants used electric blankets compared to three control infants. This was not significant (OR = 2.69 [95% CI: 0.22–23.58]).

Use of a hot water bottle

Very few of the babies ever used a hot water bottle; four SIDS infants (1.2%) and seven control infants (0.5%) used one for the last/reference sleep, a non-significant difference (OR = 2.31 [95% CI: 0.49–9.16]).

Heating in room for last/reference sleep

Assessment of heating was difficult because of the variations in heating systems, types of setting and how the setting was arranged for different rooms. Furthermore, many of the responses to 'usual practice' were dependent on outside temperature and the number of people in the house.

Data on whether the heating was on for the duration of the last sleep were gathered from the time and setting of heating, type of heating, room the baby slept in and narrative accounts. The period of the last sleep was calculated from the time the baby was last seen or heard to the time the baby was found after the sleep. For houses where the main type of heating was a night storage system, it was not assumed the heating was on, unless specifically stated. Data were obtained for 310 SIDS infants and 1,288 controls.

More SIDS (19.4%) than control infants (15.2%) slept in a room where the heating was on for at least half the duration of the last/reference sleep (OR = 1.54 [95% CI: 1.04–2.28]). For last/reference sleeps in the daytime, there was no significant difference between the proportion with the heating on for the full duration of the sleep (OR = 0.71 [95% CI: 0.29–1.65]). However, for last/reference sleeps during the night, more SIDS families had the heating on for the full duration of the sleep (OR = 1.54 [95% CI: 1.07–2.22]).

Outdoor temperatures

Information was obtained from the Meteorological Office on maximum and minimum temperatures recorded by weather stations within the study regions. The recorded temperatures for the 24-hour periods preceding the deaths and the end of the reference sleeps were obtained for the weather stations closest to the homes of the SIDS and control infants respectively. No significant difference was found in either maximum or minimum temperatures between the 24-hour period preceding the SIDS deaths and those preceding the reference sleeps. Thus, differences in heating or bedding between SIDS and controls are not accounted for by different outdoor temperatures.

How often the window was open

There was no difference between the two groups during usual night or day sleeps or for the last/reference sleep with regard to whether or not the window of the room in which the baby slept was open. Usually at night 68% of SIDS infants slept in a room where the window was never opened compared to 67.4% of control infants; during the day sleeps the proportions were 44.1% of SIDS infants and 41.2%

of controls; and for the last/reference sleep, 75.1% of SIDS infants slept in a room where the window was not open compared to 75.6% of controls (OR = 0.97 [95% CI: 0.72–1.31]).

How often the door was ajar

Significantly more of the SIDS than control infants slept in room where the door was closed for both usual night sleeps (32.3% SIDS vs. 27.3% controls, OR = 1.37 [95% CI: 1.04–1.82]) and for the last/ reference sleep (37.4% SIDS vs. 29.8% controls, OR = 1.62 [95% CI: 1.21–2.18]). For a number of infants (18 SIDS infants and 30 control infants), this question did not apply as there was either no door or the infant was sleeping outside.

Use of duvet or thick quilt

More SIDS (14.4%) than control infants (7.5%) usually slept under a duvet or a quilt both in the daytime (OR = 2.01 [95% CI: 1.41–3.08]) and at night (37.4% vs. 23.7%) (OR = 2.16 [95% CI: 1.60–2.93]). Practice on the last/reference sleep is detailed in Table 3.31.

Proportionally more SIDS infants used adult or infant duvets for the last/reference sleep. The median tog value of the adult duvets used by the SIDS infants (7.7 togs [interquartile range: 6.7–9.9 togs]) was higher than the controls (7.2 togs [interquartile range 4.5–10.2 togs]) but this was not significant ($p = 0.69$). However, the median tog values of the infant duvets used by the SIDS infants (4.9 togs [interquartile range: 3.4–7.5 togs]) was significantly higher ($p = 0.04$) than the controls (3.9 togs [interquartile range 2.3–6.7 togs]). Although most adult duvets were used while bed-sharing, and most of the infant duvets were used in a cot, this was not always the case. There was no difference in the tog value of the duvet between SIDS and control infants who spent the night in bed with a parent (median 7.8 togs for both groups). For infants who slept in a cot, however, the duvets used by SIDS infants had higher tog values (median = 6.0 togs [interquartile range: 3.5–7.6 togs]) than those used by controls (median = 3.9 togs [interquartile range: 2.3–6.3 togs]) ($p = 0.02$).

How the covers were tucked in

Having the bedding tightly tucked in for usual sleep was associated with a lower risk of SIDS at night (OR = 0.69 [95% CI: 0.48–0.98]), but, curiously, with an apparently increased risk in the daytime (OR = 1.84 [95% CI: 1.23–2.74]). More of the SIDS infants slept under loose covering for the last/ reference sleep, but this was not significant when either the use of duvets for that sleep (OR for loose covers = 0.66 [95% CI: 0.43–1.01]) or where the infant slept (OR for loose covers = 0.68 [95% CI: 0.44–1.05]) was taken into account.

Found with covers over the head

A small proportion of SIDS (4.4%) and control infants (2.7%) had on several occasions previously been found with bed covers over their heads after a sleep. A larger proportion of SIDS (16.2%) than control infants (2.9%) were found with covers over their heads after the last/reference sleep.

Of the 49 SIDS infants found with their head covered, 44 were in a cot, and of these 26 were covered by a duvet (59%). This is in marked contrast with the overall dataset, where less than a third of SIDS infants used a duvet in the cot. Of the 26 duvets, three were adult duvets. The median tog value of the remaining 23 infant duvets (6.2 tog [interquartile range: 3.6–7.6 togs] was higher than the overall median of 4.9 togs of SIDS infant duvets mentioned above. Amongst the 38 control infants found with their heads covered, 36 were in a cot and only five were covered by a duvet (median tog 4.0 [range 2.4–8 togs]).

Table 3.31 Use of duvet for last/reference sleep

	SIDS		Controls		OR (95% CI)
	n = 323	%	n = 1 299	%	
Used any duvet:					
No	195	60.4	1 034	79.6	1.00 (reference group)
Yes	128	39.6	265	20.4	2.92 (2.15–3.95)
Used infant duvet:					
No	254	78.6	1 110	85.5	1.00 (reference group)
Yes	69	21.4	189	14.5	1.85 (1.29–2.66)
Used adult duvet:					
No	264	81.7	1 223	94.1	1.00 (reference group)
Yes	59	18.3	76	5.9	3.62 (2.38–5.49)

Moving around in the bed

The present study was largely completed before the 'Feet to Foot' campaign, and we attempted to assess the effects of infants moving up or down the cot, together with the effects such movements might have on the risk of head covering.

Amongst infants who slept in cots, very few SIDS or control infants were usually put to sleep at the bottom of the cot for usual night sleeps (3.7%, 5%, respectively), day sleeps (2.4%, 2.9%, respectively), or for the last/reference sleep (2.9%, 4%, respectively). After the last/reference sleep, however, slightly more SIDS infants (8.6%) than controls (5%) were found at the bottom of the cot ($p = 0.027$, Fisher's exact test).

Concentrating on the last/reference sleep, we can specifically look at movement that may explain why infants were found with covers over their heads. 11.4% of SIDS and 4.3% of control infants had moved down the cot (from the top of the cot to the middle or bottom, or from the middle of the cot to the bottom). This difference was significant (OR = 3.51 [95% CI: 2.00–6.12]). Of the 49 SIDS infants found with covers over their heads, 24 had moved down the cot, whilst of the 38 control infants found with covers over their heads only four had moved down the cot. The risk associated with this downward movement was reduced when controlled for the head being covered, but still remained significant (OR = 2.76 [95% CI: 1.42–5.39]).

There was no difference in the proportion of SIDS and control infants put down or found against the side of the cot or the cot bumper, and no relationship between this position and the covers being found over the head.

The cot environment

Items in the cot

The word 'cot' here is used as a generic term for crib, carrycot, cradle, moses basket or any type of sleeping place made specifically for a baby to sleep in. All items in the cot except for the infant's clothes and sleeping covers are included in this analysis (e.g. soft or hard toys, pillows, cot bumpers, etc.). Items strapped to the cot such as thermometers, baby monitors and night lights are excluded, along with items hanging over the cot such as mobiles. The following analysis deals only with those infants who slept in a cot.

For usual night-time sleeps, more control infants (23.9%) than SIDS (17.6%) had three or more items in the cot ($p = 0.03$). For usual daytime sleeps, both groups had fewer items in the cot, and there was no significant difference between the groups ($p = 0.11$).

For the last/reference sleep, again more control infants (22.1%) had three or more items in the cot compared to the SIDS (19.3%), but this was not significant ($p = 0.43$). Table 3.32 shows the type of item in the cot for the usual night and day sleeps and for the last/reference sleep.

Table 3.32 Type of items in the cot

At least one of the following items	Usual night sleep				Usual day sleep				Last/reference sleep			
	SIDS		Controls		SIDS		Controls		SIDS		Controls	
	n = 256	%	n = 1 230	%	n = 209	%	n = 867	%	n = 187	%	n = 1 021	%
Pillow	18	7.0	31	2.5	15	7.2	20	2.3	17	9.1	23	2.3
Cot bumper *	57	22.3	372	30.2	39	18.7	251	29.0	49	26.2	316	31.0
Toys†	93	36.3	523	42.5	67	32.1	364	42.0	70	37.4	443	43.4

* Including 'activity bumpers', 'bolsters' and rolled-up blankets used as a bumper

† Includes all hard toys, soft toys, fabric books, play mats, etc.

Significantly more of the SIDS than control infants who slept in cots used a pillow for usual night sleeps (OR = 2.81 [95% CI: 1.48–5.28]), for usual day sleeps (OR = 3.28 [95% CI: 1.56–6.84]) and for the last/reference sleep (OR = 4.34 [95% CI: 2.17–8.67]). We do not know if the pillow was used to support the head, the whole body or was just inside the cot but not used by the infant.

More control than SIDS infants used a cot bumper for both the usual and the last/reference sleep. The difference between the two groups was associated with a significantly reduced risk for usual night sleeps (OR = 0.66 [95% CI: 0.47–0.92]) and usual day sleeps (OR = 0.56 [95% CI: 0.38–0.84]) but did not quite reach significance for the last/reference sleep (OR = 0.79 [95% CI: 0.55–1.14]).

Proportionately more of the control infants had both soft and hard toys in their cot compared to SIDS infants. With regard to the presence of a toy of any type, the difference between the two groups was not significant for usual night sleep (OR = 0.77 [95% CI: 0.5–1.03]) or for the last/reference sleep (OR = 0.78 [95% CI: 0.56–1.09]), but was associated with a significantly reduced risk for usual day sleeps (OR = 0.66 [95% CI: 0.47–0.92]).

Baby monitors

Questions about the use of various types of baby monitors were only asked in the third year of the study:

Listening devices

More of the control families sometimes or always used listening devices for both night and day sleeps, but this was not significant. For the last/reference sleep, 98 of 509 control (19.3%) and 6 of 119 SIDS (5%) families were using listening devices (OR = 0.33 [95% CI: 0.13–0.80]). Of the control families using listening devices for the reference sleep, 53% heard noises mainly described as shuffling, breathing, gurgling, crying, snoring and moaning. Of the six SIDS families using such a device, only one heard any noise, described as crying, at midnight. This infant was put down at 10.30 p.m. and was found dead at 11.30 a.m. the next morning.

Apnoea monitors

A higher proportion of SIDS (11 of 123; 8.9%) than control families (11 of 517; 2.1%) used apnoea monitors usually at night (OR = 7.72 [95% CI: 2.3–25.9]), and usually in the day (8 of 122; 6.6% SIDS vs. 12 of 510; 2.4% controls) (OR = 5.12 [95% CI: 1.58–16.79]). For the last/reference sleep the difference, although tending in the same direction, was not significant (6 of 121; 5% SIDS vs. 11 of 512; 2.1% controls) (OR = 1.17 [95% CI: 0.26–5.27]).

Baby mattress

Toxic gas theory

In 1989, Mr Barry Richardson proposed that a contributory factor in SIDS might be the production of toxic trihydride gases, arsine, stibine and phosphene by fungal degradation of flame retardants or plasticisers added to the polyvinyl chloride (PVC) of mattress covers. The hypothesis predicted that infants dying as SIDS would be more likely to be sleeping on older mattresses, those previously used by other infants and those with PVC covers. It further predicted that tissue concentrations of antimony would be higher in infants sleeping on mattresses with higher concentrations of antimony in the PVC covering material. The final prediction of the hypothesis was that if parents wrapped PVC mattresses in impermeable covers (e.g. polyethylene) the risk of SIDS would be substantially reduced. In order to investigate these hypotheses, for all three years of the study information was collected on the type, age and coverings of mattresses, and for the third year samples of mattress covers and filling were subject to mycological and chemical analyses. Also in the third year of the study, tissue and hair samples were collected from infants who died, together with hair samples from mothers of SIDS and control infants, plus hair samples from control infants.

The results of these investigations have been published in full elsewhere [7]. There was no evidence that colonisation of mattresses by the particular fungus implicated in the Richardson hypothesis (*Scopularis brevicaulis*) was common, no association between mattress concentrations of antimony and those in tissue or hair samples, and no evidence that the use of mattresses with integral PVC covers was associated with an increased risk of SIDS – in fact, the association of such mattress covers was with a significantly *lower* risk of SIDS. Higher concentrations of hair antimony in infants than in their mothers appears to represent prenatal accumulation rather than postnatal exposure. An association found in the univariate analysis between greater mattress age and the risk of SIDS was accounted for in a multivariate analysis by the lower socio-economic status and larger sibships of the SIDS infants compared with the controls. No evidence was found that wrapping mattresses in polyethylene sheeting reduced the risk of SIDS: identical proportions of SIDS and control infants slept on mattresses which had been wrapped in this way, and three SIDS deaths occurred on such wrapped mattresses.

In summary, no evidence was found to support the 'toxic gas' hypothesis.

The use of soft mattresses

Soft mattresses have been suggested as a risk factor for SIDS, particularly if infants sleep in the prone position [8]. Parents were asked to quantify how far the infant's head sank into the mattress as a measure of mattress softness. For infants who slept in a cot for the last/reference sleep, there was no significant difference between the proportion of SIDS (9.4%) and control infants (15.7%) who used a soft mattress (OR = 0.75 [95% CI: 0.47–1.20]).

Infant illness*

Apparent life-threatening event

Two questions were asked to ascertain whether any of the infants had ever experienced an apparent life-threatening event:

- Parents were asked whether the infant had ever had 'an episode in which he or she became lifeless?' This was true for 37 of 317 (11.7%) SIDS and 39 of 1,299 (3%) control infants (OR = 5.39 [95% CI: 3.11–9.34]). Of those who had experienced an episode, a similar proportion were reported to have experienced the cessation of breathing (67.6% vs. 66.6%) and a change in colour (75% vs. 81.6%), and a similar proportion had contacted a doctor (65.7% vs. 66.7%). However, more SIDS infants (43.8%) than control infants (28.2%) were reported to have had more than one episode, to have experienced apparent cessation of breathing for more than 10 seconds (55.6% vs. 21.7%) and to have been taken to hospital (47.1% vs. 33.3%).

- Parents were asked whether the infant had ever had 'any form of convulsion, fit, seizure or other turn in which consciousness was lost or any part of the body made abnormal movements?' Such events, whilst uncommon, were more frequent amongst SIDS (11 of 318; 3.5%) than control infants (12 of 1,299; 0.9%) (OR = 4.49 [95% CI: 1.80–11.17]).

Previous hospital admissions or attendances

The parents were asked whether the baby had had any hospital attendances or admissions apart from an apparent life-threatening event and the reason for admission or attendance.

More of the SIDS (28.9%) than control infants (16.6%) had had at least one admission to or attendance at hospital (OR = 2.19 [95% CI: 1.59–3.02]). The most common reasons for such attendances were SCBU follow-up (5.3% SIDS, 1.8% controls), infections (8.1%, 5.2%, respectively), accidental injury (3.4%, 1.4%, respectively), minor surgery (2.8%, 3.4%, respectively) and major surgery (2.5%, 0.5%, respectively).

The difference in hospital attendances between index and control babies remained significant (OR = 1.84 [95% CI: 1.31–2.58]) after exclusion of SCBU follow-up.

---

* This data has been published in full in *Arch. Dis. Child* (1999). See Appendix II for a full reference.

Health in the last week

Parental assessment of the infant's health

More SIDS parents than controls rated their infant's health in the last week before death or reference sleep as only fair (24.1% SIDS vs. 19.0% controls, OR = 1.45 [95% CI: 1.05–2.00]) or as poor (7.7% SIDS vs. 5.2% controls, OR = 2.18 [95% CI: 1.26–3.79]).

Medication

The parents were also asked what type of medication (including ointments, homoeopathic medicines, vitamins, etc.) the baby had been given in the last week. Whilst slightly more of the SIDS infants had been given any form of medication than had controls, this was not significant overall. Significantly more SIDS (7.4%) than control infants (1.5%) were given multivitamins, iron or folic acid (often in conjunction with each other) (OR = 5.18 [95% CI: 2.58–10.40]). However, most of these infants were extremely premature, and when adjustment was made for gestational age, vitamin and mineral intake became non-significant (OR = 1.55 [95% CI: 0.66–3.67]).

Infant seen by a health professional

More SIDS infants were seen by a health professional in the week before death (57.6%) than were controls in the week before the interview (49.6%) (OR = 1.38 [95% CI: 1.07–1.78]). However, many of these infants were apparently well and were seen for routine prearranged visits. Overall, similar proportions of SIDS (31.4%) and controls (32.1%) had been seen by a health professional in the last week, and not found to be ill. A slightly higher proportion of SIDS infants than controls had been seen by a health care professional in the last week and found to be unwell (26.1% vs. 17.5%, respectively) (OR = 1.64 [95% CI: 1.19–2.24]). The main conditions identified were infections, particularly upper respiratory infections.

Health in the last 24 hours

Parental assessment of the infant's health

More SIDS parents than controls rated their infant's health in the last 24 hours before death or reference sleep as only fair (24.9% SIDS vs. 14% controls, OR = 2.09 [95% CI: 1.49–2.93]) or poor (5.9% SIDS vs. 1.5% controls, OR = 4.83 [95% CI: 2.31–10.10]). Of those infants in both groups whose health was perceived by their parents as not good in the last 24 hours, approximately three-quarters did not have good health for the whole of that week.

Infant sweating in last 24 hours

More SIDS infants than controls had been noted by their parents to be sweating in the 24 hours before death/interview (22.1% SIDS vs. 17.2% controls, OR = 1.52 [95% CI: 1.07–2.17]), and for more of the SIDS infants than controls this was unusual (7.3% SIDS vs. 4% controls, OR = 2.10 [95% CI: 1.18–3.72]).

Feeding in last 24 hours

A similar proportion of SIDS and control infants had more feeds than usual, but significantly more of the SIDS infants than controls (13.2% vs. 5.2%) had fewer feeds than usual in the last 24 hours

(OR = 3.01 [95% CI: 1.89–4.80]. This was also reflected in a higher proportion of SIDS infants than controls who had taken a smaller volume of feed (9.1% vs. 1.5%) (OR = 7.10 [95% CI: 3.49–14.43]). As a dichotomous variable (including infants who fed more often as part of the reference group), infants feeding less frequently remained significant (OR = 3.01 [95% CI: 1.89–4.78]). As a dichotomous variable (including infants who took a slightly smaller volume than usual as part of the reference group), a reduction in the volume of feed taken remained significant (OR = 4.55 [95% CI: 2.16–9.60]).

Retrospective scoring system (Baby Check)

The Cambridge Baby Check is a scoring system to help parents and doctors quantify serious illness in babies up to six months of age. It is based on seven symptoms and 12 signs, each of which receives a score if they are evident, the higher the score the more ill the baby [3]. A retrospective version of the Baby Check, previously validated [9] was used. In this version of the scoring system, questions on infant response during the assessment could not be ascertained and parents were asked whether their infant had had a fever in the past week, instead of being asked to take the infant's temperature. The scores are grouped and action is linked to each group:

Score 0–7   Baby is generally well.
Score 8–12   Baby is unwell but not seriously ill, get health advice and observe baby.
Score 13–19   Baby is ill and needs a doctor.
Score 20+   Baby is seriously ill and needs a doctor straight away.

The maximum possible score using Baby Check is 111, and for the retrospective Baby Check is 96. Care must therefore be taken when interpreting the retrospective Baby Check results, as these will potentially underestimate the severity of ill-health in the baby.

Data were unavailable for seven SIDS infants and one control. In a few instances where mothers had failed to answer one or two items, the total score was calculated on the assumption that the sign or symptom concerned was absent. The data are summarised in Table 3.33.

Table 3.33 Composite score of retrospective Baby Check in the last 24 hours

Composite score	SIDS		Controls		OR (95% CI)
	n = 318	%	n = 1 299	%	
0–7	250	78.6	1 200	92.4	1.00 (reference group)
8–12	32	10.1	52	4.0	2.95 (1.82–4.79)
13–19	19	6.0	29	2.2	3.14 (1.67–5.91)
20+	17	5.3	18	1.4	4.53 (2.19–9.36)

The great majority of both SIDS (78.6%) and control infants (92.4%) were generally well in the 24 hours prior to the last/reference sleep. Significantly more SIDS infants were mildly unwell (score 8–12), a small but significant proportion of SIDS infants needed a doctor (score 13–19) or emergency medical attention (score 20 or more). The results are not influenced by the inclusion or exclusion of information on whether the baby had a fever in the last week. The retrospective Baby Check scores were significant if treated as a continuous variable ($p < 0.0001$).

Bed-sharing and room-sharing*

Bed-sharing

Usual habit

Table 3.34 gives the data on parents' estimates of how often they took their infant into their bed to feed, sleep or when the infant was unwell.

Table 3.34 Bed-sharing: usual practice

	SIDS		Controls		OR (95% CI)
How often to feed?	n = 317	%	n = 1 298	%	
Never	138	43.5	626	48.2	1.00 (reference group)
Rarely	39	12.3	148	11.4	1.20 (0.79–1.81)
One or two nights/week	12	3.8	49	3.8	1.11 (0.54–2.23)
More than two nights/week	16	5.0	32	2.5	2.27 (1.15–4.42)
Every night	112	35.3	443	34.1	1.15 (0.86–1.53)
How often to sleep?	n = 317	%	n = 1 299	%	
Never	134	42.3	699	53.8	1.00 (reference group)
Rarely	67	21.1	284	21.9	1.23 (0.88–1.72)
One or two nights/week	23	7.3	101	7.8	1.19 (0.71–1.98)
More than two nights/week	25	7.9	54	4.2	2.42 (1.41–4.13)
Every night	68	21.5	161	12.4	2.20 (1.55–3.13)
When unwell?	n = 315	%	n = 1 296	%	
No*	214	67.9	846	65.3	1.00 (reference group)
Yes	101	32.1	450	34.7	0.89 (0.68–1.16)

* Includes those where parent responded 'not applicable' because infant had never been unwell

A similar proportion of SIDS and control parents bed-shared for feeding or when the infant was unwell. However, significantly more SIDS parents (29%) than controls (17%) habitually slept with the infant for more than two nights a week (OR = 2.11 [95% CI: 1.54–2.89]).

---

* This data has been published in full in the *British Medical Journal* (1999). See Appendix II for details.

For last/reference sleep

Parents were asked whether they bed-shared with their infant for the last/reference sleep, and whether the infant was still in bed with the parents at the end of this sleep. A proportion of the deaths (16.9%) and reference sleeps (15.8%) occurred during the day when bed-sharing was uncommon for both groups. The results shown in the following three tables were very similar if these daytime sleeps were excluded or included, the latter option was therefore chosen. If the sleeping place was a sofa (not a sofa-bed), this was treated separately. The data are summarised in Table 3.35.

Slightly more of the SIDS infants bed-shared for at least part of the sleep, but this difference was not significant. Sharing a sofa was associated with a very high risk of SIDS; over 6% of deaths occurred whilst sleeping with an adult on a sofa (one further case where the infant was sleeping on a chair with a three year-old sibling has not been included). The narrative account suggests suffocation as the probable cause of death for at least three of these deaths. For seven of the deaths, the narrative account suggests the parents did not intend to fall asleep, whilst for another nine this practice was not unusual. For 10 of the deaths, the infant shared the sofa with the mother, for the other 10 with the father.

Table 3.35 Bed-sharing for last/reference sleep (1)

	SIDS		Controls		OR (95% CI)
	n = 321	%	n = 1 299	%	
Did not sleep with adult	195	60.7	926	71.3	1.00 (reference group)
Shared parental bed for all or part of sleep	106	33.0	367	28.3	1.25 (0.92–1.70)
Shared sofa for all or part of sleep*	20	6.2	6	0.5	20.96 (6.30–69.76)

* Two controls (none of the SIDS infants) moved from the sofa to the bed for the end of the sleep

In Table 3.36, those infants who bed-shared for part of the night but were put back in their cot and those who bed-shared for the whole night or were brought into bed and found there after the last/reference sleep have been considered separately.

Table 3.36 Bed-sharing for last/reference sleep (2)

	SIDS		Controls		OR (95% CI)
	n = 321	%	n = 1 299	%	
Did not sleep with adult	195	60.7	926	71.3	1.00 (reference group)
Bed-shared but put back in own cot	24	7.5	178	13.7	0.49 (0.29–0.81)
Found in parental bed	82	25.5	189	14.5	2.07 (1.46–2.95)
Shared sofa for all or part of sleep	20	6.2	6	0.5	22.05 (6.52–74.56)

A greater proportion of control infants bed-shared and were put back in their own cot, suggesting a protective effect. Infants who bed-shared for the whole sleep or were brought to bed for the latter part of the sleep were at increased risk. Few parents whose infant was found in the parental bed had bed-shared because the infant was unwell (1% SIDS vs. 4% controls). Similar proportions (29% SIDS vs. 29% controls) did so to feed and then fell asleep. More of the SIDS parents (44%) than controls (31%) bed-shared because they usually slept that way, and more of the control parents (31%) than SIDS (19%) because the baby would not settle. The majority of infants slept adjacent to one parent (71% SIDS vs. 59% controls), more control infants slept between parents (21% SIDS vs. 37% controls) and two SIDS infants were found under the parent. The risk associated with sofa-sharing remained highly significant.

Table 3.37 examines the relationship of both habitual parental smoking and maternal alcohol intake prior to the last/reference sleep with infants being found bed-sharing with a parent at the end of the last/reference sleep.

In 84% of the SIDS families at least one parent smoked. For those infants found in the parental bed, this proportion was 91.5 % (75 out of 82). Amongst non-smoking parents there was no identifiable risk. The possible risk associated with bed-sharing cannot therefore be generalised to the whole population. Stratification for maternal alcohol consumption before the last/reference sleep shows that a much higher proportion of bed-sharing SIDS mothers (21%) than controls (3%) consumed more than two units of alcohol.

Room-sharing

Room baby was put in for sleep

More control than SIDS infants slept in their own bedrooms, usually at night (28.3% vs. 16.1%, respectively), usually in the day (13.7% vs. 9.1%) and for the last/reference sleep (24.1% vs. 14.6%, respectively), whilst more of the SIDS infants slept in a room shared with someone other than a parent or in the lounge for the usual night sleep or last sleep. A small proportion of SIDS infants shared a room with the whole family, where this was the only room in the household. Sharing the parental bedroom (including sharing the parental bed) was more common amongst the control infants for the usual night sleep (55.9% vs. 61.2%, OR = 0.80 [95% CI: 0.58–1.12]) and for the last/reference sleep (46.7% vs. 54.6%, OR = 0.71 [95% CI: 0.5–1.00]), but these differences did not reach significance.

Who sleeps in the same room?

Significantly more of the SIDS infants (74.3% vs. 67.9%) shared a bedroom with an adult for the usual night sleep (OR = 1.40 [95% CI: 1.05–1.86), but a similar proportion (60.9% vs. 62.7%) shared the bedroom with an adult for the last/reference sleep (OR = 0.93 [95% CI: 0.72–1.20]).

Bed-sharing and room-sharing

Several mutually exclusive sleeping arrangements need to be considered:

a)   The infant slept in a room separate from an adult.

b)   The infant slept in a separate cot or bed, in a room with an adult.

c)   The infant bed-shared with an adult for part of the sleep but was then put back in a separate cot or bed.

d)   The infant bed-shared for the whole sleep or was brought to the bed for last part of sleep.

e)   The infant sofa-shared with an adult.

These possible arrangements of sleeping can be analysed as a single multicategorical variable using different groups for reference as shown in Table 3.38. The first analysis uses a) as the reference group, the second uses b) and the third again uses b) but treats categories c) and d) as one category.

Table 3.37 Found in the parental bed stratified by parental smoking and maternal alcohol consumption in the previous 24 hours

		SIDS		Controls		OR (95% CI)
At least one parent smokes	Infant found in parental bed	n = 321	%	n = 1 298	%	
No	No	44	13.7	582	44.8	1.00 (reference group)
Yes	No	195	60.7	528	40.7	5.34 (3.61–7.90)
No	Yes	7	2.2	102	7.9	1.08 (0.45–2.58)
Yes	Yes	75	23.4	86	6.6	12.35 (7.41–20.59)
Mother > 2 units alcohol	Infant found in parental bed	n = 314	%	n = 1 297	%	
No	No	213	67.8	1 074	82.8	1.00 (reference group)
Yes	No	20	6.4	35	2.7	2.63 (1.35–5.11)
No	Yes	64	20.4	182	14.0	1.82 (1.27–2.62)
Yes	Yes	17	5.4	6	0.5	14.37 (4.66–44.29)

In the first analysis, room-sharing appears to be protective if the infant does not share a bed or sofa with the parent(s). Similarly, infants who bed-shared for part of the sleep but were put back in their own bed were at less risk. Infants who bed-shared for the whole or last part of the sleep were more at risk, but this did not achieve statistical significance. Infants sharing a sofa with an adult were very much at risk.

In the second analysis, infants not room-sharing were shown to be at significant risk, as were those who bed-shared at the end of sleep, or sofa-shared. Bed-sharing for only part of the sleep showed a protective effect which did not achieve statistical significance.

In the third analysis, bed-sharing for any part of the sleep is treated as a single variable, as it could be argued, for ease of interpretation, that we do not know at what point during a bed-sharing sleep that the SIDS infants died, therefore bed-sharing for any length of time could be used as a single variable. Using this variable, bed-sharing at all remains a significant factor, whilst sleeping in a separate room remained a risk factor, and sofa-sharing remained a highly significant risk factor.

Pacifier (dummy) use*

Usual habit

There was no identifiable difference in the frequency of use of a pacifier between SIDS and control infants at night-time (61% SIDS and 60.5% controls, OR = 1.03 [95% CI: 0.78–1.36]) or in daytime sleeps (66.4% SIDS, 65.5% controls, OR = 1.04 [95% CI: 0.78–1.38]).

---

* This data has been published in full in the *Archives of Diseases in Childhood* (1999). See Appendix II for a full reference.

Table 3.38 Room-sharing and bed-sharing with an adult (mutually exclusive groups)

	SIDS		Controls		OR (95% CI)
	n = 321	%	n = 1 299	%	
Analysis 1					
Did not room-share	114	35.5	420	32.3	1.00 (reference group)
Room-shared only (not bed-share)	81	25.2	506	39.0	0.50 (0.35–0.73)
*Bed-shared, but not by end of sleep**	24	7.5	178	13.7	0.34 (0.20–0.59)
Bed-shared all or at end of sleep	82	25.5	189	14.5	1.41 (0.93–2.12)
Sofa-shared†	20	6.2	6	0.5	16.07 (4.55–56.72)
Analysis 2					
Room-shared only (non-bed-share)	81	25.2	506	39.0	1.00 (reference group)
Did not room-share	114	35.5	420	32.3	1.92 (1.32–2.80)
Bed-shared, but not by end of sleep	24	7.5	178	13.7	0.66 (0.38–1.13)
Bed-shared all or at end of sleep	82	25.5	189	14.5	2.75 (1.85–4.08)
Sofa-shared	20	6.2	6	0.5	31.25 (8.78–111.23)
Analysis 3					
Room-shared only (non-bed-share)	81	25.2	506	39.0	1.00 (reference group)
Did not room-share	114	35.5	420	32.3	1.96 (1.34–2.85)
Bed-shared for at least part of sleep	106	33.0	367	28.3	1.67 (1.17–2.39)
Sofa-shared	20	6.2	6	0.5	29.97 (8.54–105.19)

* Twelve SIDS and 39 controls then put back in own room, the rest put back in parental bedroom

† Two controls did not share the sofa by the end of the sleep

Habitual pacifier use was more common in families from social class V and those who were unemployed, for both SIDS and controls (81.4% and 82.8%, respectively), and less common amongst those in classes I and II (53.1% and 57.8%, respectively), but there were no significant differences in pacifier use between SIDS and controls within any single social class.

At time of last/reference sleep

Significantly more of the control infants were given a pacifier for the reference sleep (51.2%), compared with SIDS infants for their last sleep (39.6%) (OR = 0.62 [95% CI: 0.46–0.83]).

Table 3.39 shows the relationship between habitual pacifier use and use for the last/reference sleep.

Table 3.39 Comparison of usual pacifier use and use for the last/reference sleep

Usually used a pacifier	Used pacifier for last/reference sleep	SIDS		Controls		OR (95% CI)	Bivariate OR (95% CI)*
		n = 313	%	n = 1 296	%		
No	No	95	30.4	386	29.8	1.00 (reference group)	1.00 (reference group)
Yes	No	94	30.0	246	19.0	1.55 (1.11–2.18)	1.39 (0.93–2.07)
No	Yes	5	1.6	36	2.8	0.56 (0.17–1.50)	0.37 (0.10–1.20)
Yes	Yes	119	38.0	628	48.5	0.77 (0.57–1.05)	0.63 (0.44–0.91)

* Controlling for socio-economic status using occupational classification

The use of a pacifier for the last/reference sleep was protective, but not significantly so. However, babies who usually used a pacifier but did not do so for the last/reference sleep were at significantly greater risk, although this risk loses significance after socio-economic status is taken into account.

The apparent protective effect of pacifier use for the last sleep seems to arise from the fact that there was a higher proportion of SIDS infants who normally used a pacifier but did not do so for their last sleep.

Breast-feeding

Table 3.40 shows the prevalence and duration of breast-feeding for SIDS and control infants. Significantly more of the control mothers had attempted to breastfeed. However, there was no identifiable dose-response effect with increasing duration of breast-feeding. If the 16 SIDS and 27 control infants who were less than four weeks old are excluded from the group who breast-fed longest, there is little change in the degree of significance (OR = 0.44 [95% CI: 0.32–0.59]).

Pattern of previous sleep

Length of previous sleep

The parents were asked to recall the longest period for which their baby had slept in the 24 hours before the last or reference sleep. The median longest sleep for the index infants was 6 hours and 10 minutes (interquartile range: 3 hours 45 minutes to 8 hours 40 minutes) compared to 7 hours 20 minutes (interquartile range: 5 hours to 9 hours 50 minutes] for the controls. As a continuous variable this was significant ($p < 0.0001$).

Table 3.41 compares the distribution of relatively short and long sleeps.

Significantly more of the SIDS infants slept for shorter periods, and significantly more control infants slept for longer periods. A similar proportion of SIDS and control parents thought the length of the longest sleep was the same as usual (SIDS: 72.2% vs. controls: 73.5%), longer than usual (SIDS: 15.4% vs. controls: 15.2%), or shorter than usual (SIDS: 12.4% vs. controls: 10.9%). For the subgroup of infants whose longest period of sleep was four hours or less in the previous 24 hours, 17% of parents from both groups thought this sleep was shorter than usual.

How many times the baby woke

The question was asked as to how many times the baby woke in the sleep immediately prior to the last/ reference sleep, and whether this was usual. A similar proportion of SIDS (38.6%) and controls (36.1%) did not wake during this sleep, woke once (25.5%, 30.5%, respectively), twice (25.2%, 22.4%, respectively), or more often (10.7%, 10.9%, respectively). A similar large majority of both groups thought that the number of awakenings was usual (SIDS: 86.8% vs. controls: 84.2%).

Table 3.40 Prevalence and duration of breast-feeding

	SIDS		Controls		OR (95% CI)
	n = 323	%	n = 1 298	%	
Ever breast-fed					
No	182	56.3	524	40.4	1.00 (reference group)
Yes	141	43.7	774	59.6	0.47 (0.35–0.62)
Dose-response					
Never breast-fed	182	56.3	524	40.4	1.00 (reference group)
≤ 1 week	23	7.1	107	8.2	0.47 (0.27–0.81)
> 1 week ≤ 4 weeks	27	8.4	144	11.1	0.61 (0.38–0.98)
> 4 weeks*	91	28.2	523	40.3	0.43 (0.31–0.60)

* Includes 16 SIDS and 27 controls < 4 weeks but were still breast-feeding up to last/reference sleep

Table 3.41 Length of longest sleep in previous 24 hours

Length of previous sleep	SIDS		Controls		OR (95% CI)
	n = 303	%	n = 1 297	%	
5–10 hours	176	58.1	803	61.9	1.00 (reference group)
Less than 5 hours	87	28.7	192	14.8	1.99 (1.39–2.84)
More than 10 hours	40	13.2	302	23.3	0.49 (0.32–0.75)

Maternal postnatal depression

The mother was asked whether she had suffered or was still suffering from postnatal depression, and whether she thought that either her own health visitor or general practitioner believed that she was suffering from postnatal depression. An assessment of the severity of the depression perceived by health care professionals was also taken from the records made by the health visitor *prior* to the index infant's death or the interview with the control family.

Mothers in both groups more commonly thought that they were suffering or had suffered from postnatal depression than did the relevant health care professionals.

More SIDS (20.1%) than control mothers (17.4%) felt that they were suffering or had suffered from postnatal depression, but this was not statistically significant (OR = 1.19 [95% CI: 0.86–1.65]). More SIDS (10.3%) than control mothers (5.9%) thought that their general practitioner had recognised their postnatal depression (OR = 1.92 [95% CI: 1.11–3.32]). There was no significant difference between the proportion of SIDS (9.9%) and control (7.3%) mothers who thought their health visitor had recognised the problem.

From the health visitor records, mild postnatal depression had more commonly been identified amongst control (12.2%) than SIDS mothers (9.6%), although this was not statistically significant. Severe postnatal depression was rarely observed but was significantly more common amongst SIDS (2.2%) than control mothers (0.8%) (OR = 3.46 [95% CI: 1.13–10.48]).

Recent major life events

Moving accommodation in the last year

Over twice as many of the SIDS (47.1%) as control families (21%) had moved home at least once in the previous year (OR = 3.39 [95% CI: 2.53–4.55]). Families reported having moved home from between none and eight times. These results are detailed in Table 3.42.

The risk associated with moving accommodation in the last year rose with the number of moves, regardless of whether before or after the infant's birth. The risk associated with moving at least once before (OR = 3.04 [95% CI: 2.12–4.17]) or after the birth of the infant (OR = 3.76 [95% CI: 2.39–5.92]) was similar.

Changes in family routine ·

The parents were asked whether the main carer (usually the parents) had had any change in routine which would involve the infant in the 48 hours before the index infant's death or the time of the interview for the controls. The changes identified were similar in both groups, and included going out for the first time in a while; visiting friends; going on holiday; shopping or going out socialising. Significantly more index (20.6%) than control carers (12.7%) reported a perceived significant change in routine (OR = 1.97 [95% CI: 1.35–2.87]).

Air travel

Only two infants had travelled by air in the previous month. Both were control infants and both were for family skiing trips to the mountains. A further control infant had made a journey by air, but not in the previous month. No SIDS infant in this study had ever been in an aeroplane or made a trip to high altitude.

Table 3.42 Number of moves of accommodation in the last year

Number of moves in the last year:	SIDS		Controls		OR (95% CI)
	n = 323	%	n = 1 297	%	
None	171	52.9	1 024	79.0	1.00 (reference group)
One	100	31.0	219	16.9	2.74 (1.98–3.78)
Two	29	9.0	34	2.6	5.37 (2.92–9.85)
Three or more	23	7.1	20	1.5	8.38 (3.99–17.62)
Before the birth:					
None	204	63.2	1 080	83.3	1.00 (reference group)
One	85	26.3	180	13.9	2.53 (1.79–3.58)
Two or more	34	10.5	37	2.9	5.84 (3.29–10.38)
After the birth:					
None	268	83.0	1 217	93.8	1.00 (reference group)
One	42	13.0	73	5.6	3.21 (1.97–5.22)
Two or more	13	4.0	7	0.5	9.48 (3.17–28.33)

Smoking*

Maternal smoking

The mother was asked what type of cigarettes she smoked at the time of interview. Significantly more SIDS (74.0%) than control (31.3%) mothers smoked (OR = 6.21 [95% CI: 4.68–8.25]). More control mothers smoked filtered cigarettes, whilst more SIDS mothers smoked higher tar and non-filtered cigarettes.

Table 3.43 gives details of the mothers' smoking habits before, during and after pregnancy.

The majority of mothers (86.4% SIDS vs. 88.7% controls) maintained the same habit of smoking or non-smoking before, during and after pregnancy.

---

* Data from the first two years has been published in full in the *British Medical Journal* (1996). See Appendix II for a full reference.

Table 3.43 Maternal smoking before, during and after pregnancy

Before pregnancy	During pregnancy	After pregnancy	SIDS n = 322	%	Controls n = 1 299	%
Non-smoker	Non-smoker	Non-smoker	81	25.2	845	65.1
Smoker	Non-smoker	Non-smoker	9	2.8	50	3.8
Non-smoker	Smoker	Non-smoker	0	0	0	0
Non-smoker	Non-smoker	Smoker	5	1.6	8	0.6
Smoker	Smoker	Non-smoker	14	4.3	36	2.8
Smoker	Non-smoker	Smoker	15	4.7	48	3.7
Non-smoker	Smoker	Smoker	1	0.3	5	0.4
Smoker	Smoker	Smoker	197	61.2	307	23.6

Tables 3.44–3.46 show the risk associated with maternal smoking before, during and after pregnancy, along with the dose-response relationship of the risk associated with the number of cigarettes smoked.

Table 3.44 Maternal smoking before pregnancy and dose-response effect

	SIDS n = 322	%	Controls n = 1 299	%	OR (95% CI)
Non-smoker	87	27.0	858	66.1	1.00 (reference group)
Smoker before pregnancy	235	73.0	441	33.9	5.83 (4.23–8.04)
Number of cigarettes:					
Non-smoker	87	27.0	858	66.1	1.00 (reference group)
1–9 cigarettes	49	15.2	138	10.6	4.09 (2.60–6.42)
10–19 cigarettes	107	33.2	188	14.5	6.18 (4.21–9.09)
20–29 cigarettes	60	18.6	96	7.4	7.12 (4.67–11.06)
30+ cigarettes	19	5.9	19	1.5	

Table 3.45 Maternal smoking during pregnancy and dose-response effect

	SIDS		Controls		OR (95% CI)
	n = 322	%	n = 1 299	%	
Non-smoker	110	34.2	951	73.2	1.00 (reference group)
Smoker during pregnancy	212	65.8	348	26.8	5.59 (4.10–7.64)
Number of cigarettes:					
Non-smoker	110	34.2	951	73.2	1.00 (reference group)
1–9 cigarettes	87	27.0	186	14.3	4.25 (2.93–6.18)
10–19 cigarettes	75	23.3	110	8.5	6.49 (4.23–9.96)
20–29 cigarettes	34	10.6	37	2.8	} 8.56
30+ cigarettes	16	5.0	15	1.2	(5.12–14.31)

Table 3.46 Maternal smoking after pregnancy and dose-response effect

	SIDS		Controls		OR (95% CI)
	n = 322	%	n = 1 299	%	
Non-smoker	104	32.3	931	71.7	1.00 (reference group)
Smoker after pregnancy	218	67.7	368	28.3	5.95 (4.34–8.15)
Number of cigarettes:					
Non-smoker	104	32.3	931	71.7	1.00 (reference group)
1–9 cigarettes	86	26.7	158	12.2	5.30 (3.61–7.78)
10–19 cigarettes	71	22.0	145	11.2	5.25 (3.44–8.01)
20–29 cigarettes	43	13.4	54	4.2	} 8.53
30+ cigarettes	18	5.6	11	0.8	(5.33–13.67)

There was a strong dose-response effect, the more the mother smoked before, during and after pregnancy the greater the associated risk of SIDS to the baby.

Paternal smoking

Table 3.47 shows the risk associated with the smoking habits of the partner and the dose-response effect.

Table 3.47 Smoking habits of partner and dose-response effect

	SIDS		Controls		OR (95% CI)
	n = 322	%	n = 1 298	%	
Partner did not smoke*	115	35.7	827	63.7	1.00 (reference group)
Partner smoked	207	64.3	471	36.3	3.60 (2.68–4.83)
Number of cigarettes:					
Non-smoker	115	35.7	827	63.7	1.00 (reference group)
1–9 cigarettes	53	16.5	164	12.6	2.75 (1.80–4.19)
10–19 cigarettes	90	28.0	188	14.5	3.81 (2.65–5.48)
20–29 cigarettes	50	15.5	97	7.5	} 4.32
30+ cigarettes	14	4.3	22	1.7	(2.87–6.51)

* Includes mothers without partners

More partners of mothers of SIDS infants smoked than did those of control mothers. There was also a dose-response effect.

Other people smoking in the household

Table 3.48 gives information on smokers other than mothers and their partners who also lived in the same households.

Although the numbers are small, there appears to be a dose-response effect.

Table 3.48 Smoking habits of others in the household and dose-response effect

	SIDS		Controls		OR (95% CI)
	n = 322	%	n = 1 298	%	
No other smoker	281	87.3	1 222	94.1	1.00 (reference group)
Other smoker in household*	41	12.7	76	5.9	2.49 (1.56–3.96)
Number of cigarettes:					
Non-smoker	281	87.3	1 222	94.1	1.00 (reference group)
1–9 cigarettes	8	2.5	23	1.8	1.80 (0.70–4.62)
10–19 cigarettes	15	4.7	27	2.1	2.14 (1.03–4.44)
20–29 cigarettes	11	3.4	20	1.5	} 3.40
30+ cigarettes	7	2.2	6	0.5	(1.69–6.83)

* Excluding mothers and partners

Postnatal exposure

Maternal smoking after pregnancy is not an accurate proxy measure of infant postnatal exposure, because it does not take into account smoking by partners and others in the household, whether smoking was allowed in the same room as the infant or exposure outside the household. We asked parents to estimate the number of hours each day that the infant spent in a smoky atmosphere in order to assess total postnatal exposure to tobacco smoke. Information was also collected on the number of smokers in the household, the number of cigarettes they smoked, and whether smoking was allowed in the same room as the infant.

Number of smokers and cigarettes smoked in the household

Table 3.49 gives the total number of smokers in each household.

Table 3.49 Number of smokers in the household and dose-response effect

	SIDS		Controls		OR (95% CI)
	n = 321	%	*n = 1 298*	%	
No smokers	43	13.4	661	50.9	1.00 (reference group)
At least one smoker*	278	86.6	637	49.1	7.30 (4.99–10.68)
Number of smokers:					
None	43	13.4	661	50.9	1.00 (reference group)
One	103	32.1	360	27.7	4.67 (3.07–7.09)
Two	151	47.0	247	19.0	11.34 (7.37–17.44)
Three	20	6.2	28	2.2	} 16.88
Four	4	1.2	2	0.2	(7.92–35.99)

* Including mothers, partner and others

At the time of interview, at least one person smoked in 86.6% of the index households compared to 49.1% of the control households. The risk increased as the number of smokers increased.

Table 3.50 shows the dose-response effect, in terms of the average number of cigarettes smoked by all the smokers in the household.

Smoking when the infant was present

Significantly more parents of SIDS infants (48.8%) than of control infants (21.2%) permitted people to smoke in the same room as the infant (OR = 4.10 [95% CI: 3.01–5.58]). The risk associated with this practice rose with increasing numbers of smokers in the household, from just under a threefold risk (OR = 2.83 [95% CI: 1.66–4.70]) for families in which there was one smoker, to more than a sixfold risk (OR = 6.59 [95% CI: 2.97–14.64]) when there were three or more smokers.

Table 3.51 shows the average number of cigarettes smoked by all smokers for those households where smoking was allowed in the same room as the infant. There was a strong dose-response effect (although it cannot be assumed that the infant was present when all these cigarettes were smoked).

Table 3.50 Number of cigarettes smoked in the household

Number of cigarettes	SIDS		Controls		OR (95% CI)
	n = 321	%	n = 1 298	%	
None	43	13.4	661	50.9	1.00 (reference group)
1–19 cigarettes	91	28.3	330	25.4	4.40 (2.86–6.77)
20–39 cigarettes	109	34.0	209	16.1	9.31 (5.98–14.51)
40–59 cigarettes	53	16.5	74	5.7	13.98 (8.07–24.22)
60 or more cigarettes	25	7.8	24	1.8	18.64 (8.75–39.70)

Table 3.51 Number of cigarettes smoked in households where smoking was allowed with the infant present

Number of cigarettes	SIDS		Controls		OR (95% CI)
	n = 320	%	n = 1 296	%	
None	165	51.6	1 046	80.7	1.00 (reference group)
1–19 cigarettes	31	9.7	88	6.8	2.80 (1.66–4.70)
20–39 cigarettes	65	20.3	102	7.9	4.62 (3.03–7.02)
40–59 cigarettes	39	12.2	46	3.5	6.35 (3.72–10.85)
60 or more cigarettes	20	6.3	14	1.1	10.41 (4.60–23.52)

Parental estimate of infant's daily exposure to tobacco smoke

As a more direct measure of the infant's postnatal tobacco smoke exposure, we also asked the parents to estimate on an average day approximately how many hours the baby was exposed to a smoky atmosphere. This included exposure outside, as well as inside, the household (Table 3.51).

The results in Table 3.52 may slightly underestimate the prevalence and risk of smoking, because for 29 households (17 SIDS and 12 controls), all but one of which were smoking households, the parents failed to answer this question. Furthermore, some of the non-respondents found it difficult to give an estimate, whilst others claimed that because they 'blew the smoke away from the baby' or 'always opened the window' that their infant was never exposed.

There was a clear dose-response effect: the more hours of exposure, the greater the associated risk. As a continuous variable, daily exposure to tobacco smoke was significant ($p < 0.0001$).

Table 3.52 Parental estimation of infant's daily exposure to tobacco smoke

	SIDS		Controls		OR (95% CI)
	n = 308	%	n = 1 288	%	
No exposure	143	46.4	990	76.9	1.00 (reference group)
At least one hour of exposure	165	53.6	298	23.1	4.37 (3.20–5.97)
Number of hours:					
0 hours	143	46.4	990	76.9	1.00 (reference group)
1–2 hours	43	14.0	137	10.6	2.43 (1.53–3.86)
3–5 hours	33	10.7	72	5.6	3.84 (2.23–6.61)
6–8 hours	29	9.4	34	2.6	5.89 (3.19–10.86)
> 8 hours	60	19.5	55	4.3	8.30 (4.94–13.95)

Alcohol and illegal substance use

Maternal alcohol consumption

Before pregnancy

The mother was asked how much alcohol she consumed before the pregnancy in an average week.

Table 3.53 uses weekly consumption of 1–10 alcohol units as the reference group and looks at the risk associated with having a mother who drank no alcohol or one who drank more than 10 units a week (approximately 75% of the recommended maximum weekly average intake for women).

Table 3.53 Weekly maternal alcohol consumption before pregnancy

Units per week	SIDS		Controls		OR (95% CI)
	n = 309	%	n = 1 296	%	
1–10 units a week	108	35.0	638	49.2	1.00 (reference group)
Less than 1 unit	161	52.1	567	43.8	1.76 (1.30–2.38)
> 10 units a week	40	12.9	91	7.0	2.32 (1.44–3.73)

The usual alcohol consumption habits of the SIDS mothers before pregnancy was more likely to be at either end of the range in that significantly more SIDS mothers either drank no alcohol or drank more than 10 units a week. For those mothers who drank more than 10 units of alcohol a week, the median number of units consumed by the index mothers was 20 units a week (interquartile range: 14–31 units), compared to 15 units consumed by the control mothers (interquartile range: 12–19 units).

During pregnancy

Mothers were asked how their alcohol intake had changed during pregnancy. More than 98% of both SIDS and control mothers who drank less than one unit of alcohol per week before pregnancy did not drink alcohol at all during pregnancy. The majority of SIDS (85.2%) and control mothers (87.3%) who usually drank 1–10 units per week decreased their alcohol consumption during pregnancy (57% SIDS and 58% control mothers in this group giving up completely).

Within the group of heavier drinkers, more control (91.2%) than SIDS mothers (82.5%) decreased their alcohol consumption (Fisher's exact test: $p = 0.23$).

After pregnancy

Alcohol consumption after pregnancy was asked for in relation to changes from the level of consumption before pregnancy.

After pregnancy, a small proportion of mothers in both groups who had not usually drunk alcohol before pregnancy began to do so (6.2% SIDS mothers, 7.5% controls). Of those mothers who had formerly drunk 1–10 units, proportionally more of the SIDS than control mothers (20.4% vs. 11.7%, respectively) increased their consumption. This difference was significant (OR = 1.97 [95% CI: 1.12–3.43]). Of those mothers who had formerly drunk more than 10 units, 76.9% of the control mothers decreased their alcohol consumption compared to 52.5% of the SIDS mothers. Again, this was a significant difference (OR = 3.02 [95% CI: 1.28–7.17]). Overall, any increase in the level of alcohol consumption from before to after pregnancy was associated with an increased risk of SIDS (OR = 1.57 [95% CI: 1.05–2.33]).

Binge drinking

Mothers were asked how many times in an average week after pregnancy they would consume more than four units of alcohol in any one session. Significantly more SIDS (6.4%) than control mothers (1.3%) had two or more sessions per week in which they consumed more than four units of alcohol (OR = 5.54 [95% CI: 2.43–12.62]).

Drinking in the 24 hours before the last sleep

More control (13%) than SIDS mothers (7.7%) had one or two units of alcohol in the 24 hours before the last/reference sleep, but significantly more of the SIDS (15.1%) than control mothers (3.2%) had three units or more (OR = 3.97 [95% CI: 2.30–6.86]). As a continuous variable, significantly more of the index mothers consumed alcohol ($p < 0.0001$) in this time period.

Overall pattern of maternal alcohol consumption

In conclusion, there was a consistent difference between the SIDS and control mothers in terms of both the quantity and the patterns of their alcohol consumption. More SIDS mothers drank heavily before pregnancy, and fewer of them reduced their intake during and after pregnancy. More mothers of SIDS infants had a pattern of alcohol intake characterised by many units on a few occasions, whilst for control mothers the pattern was more commonly of a few units on many occasions. Significantly more index mothers drank relatively large amounts of alcohol in the 24 hours preceding the death of their infant than did control mothers in the 24 hours preceding the interview.

Alcohol consumption of partner

Weekly consumption

The mothers' partners were also asked about their alcohol intake. The median weekly alcohol intake for the partners of mothers of both SIDS and control infants was four units [interquartile range: 0–16 units and 0–12 units, respectively]. More of the control partners drank between one and 15 units a week, whilst more of the SIDS partners consumed either no alcohol or more than 15 units. As a continuous variable, usual weekly alcohol consumption between the SIDS and control partners was significantly different ($p = 0.02$). The partners' weekly alcohol intake is shown in Table 3.54. As in Table 3.53, the cut-off between the upper and middle groups is approximately 75% of the recommended maximum weekly intake.

Table 3.54 Weekly alcohol consumption of mothers' partners

Units per week	SIDS		Controls		OR (95% CI)
	n = 269	%	n = 1 230	%	
1–15 units a week	101	37.5	643	52.3	1.00 (reference group)
Less than 1 unit	100	37.2	376	30.6	1.95 (1.37–2.78)
> 15 units a week	68	25.3	211	17.2	2.15 (1.46–3.18)

Binge drinking

Significantly more SIDS (21.6%) than control partners (14.2%) had two or more sessions per week in which they consumed more than four units of alcohol (OR = 1.60 [95% CI: 1.10–2.34]).

Drinking in the 24 hours before the last sleep

As a continuous variable, the alcohol consumption of the SIDS and control partners in the 24 hours preceding the last/reference sleep was not significantly different ($p = 0.11$). More SIDS (24/292: 8.2%) than control partners (44/1,256: 3.5%) consumed seven or more units in the 24 hours before the last/reference sleep (OR = 1.90 [95% CI: 1.06–3.41]).

Overall pattern of alcohol intake by the mother's partner

Similar to the mothers of SIDS infants, their partners' intakes of alcohol, both usual and in the past 24 hours, was characterised by a higher prevalence of complete abstainers and those with a 'binge' pattern of intake.

Maternal use of illegal substance

The mothers were asked whether in the year before pregnancy, during or after pregnancy they had used any of the listed illegal substances (glue, amphetamines, barbiturates, cannabis, speed, LSD, cocaine, ecstasy, methadone, heroin, crack) on more than one occasion.

A higher proportion of SIDS (15.9%) than control mothers (5.6%), had used one or more of these illegal drugs on more than one occasion before pregnancy, during pregnancy (8.3% vs. 1.5%) and after pregnancy

(8.6% vs. 2.6%). The differences were statistically significant (before pregnancy – OR = 3.55 [95% CI: 2.24–5.61]; during pregnancy – OR = 6.88 [95% CI: 3.17–14.93]; after pregnancy – OR = 4.52 [95% CI: 2.37–8.65]). The drug most commonly used was cannabis.

Partner's use of illegal substance

The partners were asked whether they had taken any of the same listed substances on more than one occasion.

Similar to the SIDS mothers, a higher proportion of their partners (57/285: 20%) than of control partners (85/1,259: 6.8%) had tried at least one substance more than once in the year before the pregnancy and since the beginning of the pregnancy (14.8% vs. 4.5%). Both differences were statistically significant (before pregnancy – OR = 3.68 [95% CI: 2.38–5.69]; after pregnancy – OR = 4.54 [95% CI: 2.64–7.80]). Again, the drug most commonly used was cannabis. Including single mothers in the reference group (in the sense that the infant is not exposed to such a factor) the risk remained significant (before pregnancy – OR = 3.60 [95% CI: 2.35–5.53]; after pregnancy – OR = 4.50 [95% CI: 2.64–7.66]).

Non-parental care in last 24 hours

Parents were asked whether the baby had been in the care of someone other than the parents at any time in the last 24 hours. Five SIDS infants were excluded because they were in hospital during the last 24 hours. Proportionally more of the SIDS infants were under the supervision of someone other than the parents for some part of the last 24 hours (21% SIDS vs. 17.4% controls), but this difference was not significant (OR = 1.26 [95% CI: 0.92–1.74]). Significantly more of the SIDS infants were looked after by a babysitter (15 of 321 (4.7%) SIDS vs. 11 of 1,299 (0.8%) controls, OR = 4.86 [95% CI: 2.07–11.42]) in the last 24 hours, although none of the SIDS deaths occurred whilst under the supervision of the babysitter. There was no clear pattern of duration of non-parental care. Slightly more of the SIDS infants were in the care of others for more than two hours, but this difference was not significant (OR = 1.31 [95% CI: 0.89–1.93]).

Immunisations

Immunisation details (*Haemophilus influenzae* type B, oral polio and diphtheria, tetanus and pertussis) were recorded in the parent-held record for 93% of SIDS infants and 95% of controls. The recommended national immunisation programme at the time of this study was for all three immunisations to be given at two, three, and four months of age. Of the control infants, 66.6% had begun or had completed their immunisation programme, compared with 48.8% of the SIDS. In a univariate comparison, taking age into account, this difference is highly significant (OR = 0.23 [95% CI: 0.14–0.37]) and is not affected by controlling for socio-economic status or maternal smoking during pregnancy.

For those infants who had commenced their immunisation programme, the median age and the interquartile range of ages at which the first immunisation was given were virtually the same for the SIDS and controls (SIDS – 60 days [interquartile range: 56–70 days]; controls – 59 days [interquartile range: 55–63 days]); 97% had received their first injection by 90 days of age. Of the 155 SIDS infants and 412 control infants who had not started the programme, 29 SIDS and 50 controls were aged 90 days or more. If these older infants are regarded as potential 'refusers of immunisation' and compared to those who began or completed the immunisation programme, the apparent protective effect of immunisation remains (OR = 0.26 [95% CI: 0.14–0.50]).

The median time from last immunisation to interview or death was similar in the two groups (SIDS – 28 days [interquartile range: 16–68 days]; controls – 29 days [interquartile range: 13–70 days]). Table 3.55 breaks down this time interval.

As a continuous variable, the difference in the time interval was not significant ($p = 0.78$). In the 48 hours before death, 7 out of 303 SIDS infants (2.3%) were immunised compared to 41 out of 1,234 control infants (3.3%) in the 48 hours before the reference sleep.

There was thus no evidence that recent immunisation was associated with an increased risk of SIDS, and indeed the data suggest that immunisation may have a protective effect against SIDS.

Table 3.55 Time between last immunisation and death or interview

Time interval between last immunisation and death or parental interview	SIDS		Controls	
	n = 148	%	n = 822	%
0–7 days	17	11.5	119	14.5
8–14 days	14	9.5	104	12.7
15–21 days	25	16.9	99	12.0
22–28 days	19	12.8	80	9.7
29–35 days	5	3.4	58	7.1
> 35 days	68	45.9	362	44.0

% denominator is of the total infants who began programme

SIDS: MULTIVARIATE MODELS OF RISK FACTORS

Conditional multiple logistic regression

The questions collated in this study were specifically based on the knowledge of SIDS risk factors at the time the study was planned. Hence, many of these factors would be expected to be significant in the univariate analysis. These findings cannot be considered as single entities, as they do not occur in isolation but in association with many other factors. In order to understand these complex interactions, variations in several factors need to be studied simultaneously, using the techniques of multivariate analysis. The models used in this analysis were based on a single dependent outcome variable (whether the infant died as SIDS, or was a control) and two or more explanatory predictor variables. The risk associated with each predictor variable was calculated using *conditional multiple logistic regression*. This technique stems from basic linear *regression*, where the value of one variable can be predicted from the value of the other. The outcome variable was binary (that is, whether the infant died or survived), hence the term *logistic*, and as there were several predictor variables the regression analysis was termed *multiple logistic regression*. The data in this study were also matched in that control infants were matched as closely as possible to the age of the index (SIDS) infants. The regression was therefore *conditional* on the matching, the age distribution was taken into account for each model and the results were conditional on the fact that the two groups were of similar age.

Entry criteria for multivariate models

To choose which variables were allowed in the multivariate model, entry criteria needed to be adopted before the analysis began. The variables to be tested were chosen using the following criteria:

- The variable must directly relate to one of the primary hypotheses or epidemiological characteristics set out before the study began.

- In the univariate analysis, the variable must have achieved statistical significance ($p < 0.05$). Significance levels chosen for inclusion of factors in multivariate models are commonly less stringent than this (for example: $p < 0.10$, $p < 0.15$ or $p < 0.20$), as the adverse or protective effects of some univariate factors may become more significant when other variables are added to the model. However, for this study, with so many variables being investigated, a stricter criterion was set to reduce the possibility of false-positive findings from chance.

- If more than 5% of values were missing, the variable was initially treated separately from the modelling process. Although many variables had values from only one or two infants missing, this became a cumulative effect when many variables were added to the model. Those variables for which many values were missing were therefore excluded from this earlier process and tested later once the best fitting models were finalised.

- For some variables, it was difficult to identify which of the many possible indicators were the most appropriate to use. For instance, there were several indicators for socio-economic deprivation, some of which may be so closely correlated that one proxy measure would be sufficient for the analysis. For these variables, an initial investigation was conducted before the modelling process began.

Variable selection

There are four main approaches to automatic selection procedures, none of which provide infallible tactics in producing predictor variables. The *forward* procedure begins with a null model and adds each significant variable until the addition of a further variable is (in some sense) insignificant, the disadvantage being that variables included in the final model may have only been significant in the early stages of the procedure. The *backward* procedure is similar but starts with a full model and eliminates the least significant, the disadvantage being that variables may be eliminated at an early stage but may have proved significant in the later stages. The *stepwise* procedure overcomes both these disadvantages by using the forward procedure but allowing elimination as in the backward procedure. Finally, there is the *best-subset selection* procedure which calculates the best fitting model for any given number of predictor variables, although individual variables may not be significant.

For this analysis, the stepwise procedure was used. These procedures are a useful exploratory device but do not produce a definitive multivariate model that will answer all the hypotheses. For this we need to structure several different models using an intuitive approach with careful interpretation of variables that remain or fall out of the model.

Models and multivariate techniques

Several conditional multiple logistic regression models and different multivariate techniques were utilised to help interpret the complex relationships between different factors. These included:

- a two-stage empirical model described below;

- a temporal model in which the factors associated with SIDS are added sequentially, in the time order in which they would be likely to occur. In this model, the initial factors included are those present at the time of conception, followed by those relating to pregnancy, those identifiable at birth; postnatal factors are added after this, and finally those factors relating to the circumstances just before the last/reference sleep;

- factor-specific models based on restricting entry criteria using a priori knowledge of known confounders and co-factors that may have a plausible relationship with the factor under investigation;

- subgroup analysis using all of the above methods but investigating particular subgroups such as younger or older infants;

- bivariate stratification to test for consistency of one factor within different strata of another factor;

- multicategorical testing of certain factors where possible to test for a biological or dose-response relationship;

- logistical regression to test directly any differences between SIDS infants and the explained deaths presented in the section 'Explained SUDI';

- utilisation of the Wald score to construct predictor variables to identify 'high risk' families.

Using these techniques for this or any other study will not provide definitive answers to the hypotheses raised but could, with careful interpretation, if used in conjunction with univariate data and results of previous studies, lead to some tentative conclusions. To give some insight into the process of how these models are constructed and the difficulties of interpreting the results, the two-stage empirical model is outlined below.

The two-stage empirical model and its limitations

This model attempts to utilise all the factors, the only entry criteria being that factors were significant at the 5% level in the univariate analysis and less than 5% of the data were missing for each factor. Some factors describe the variation between the cases and controls but were not themselves amenable to change. These have been termed epidemiological characteristics and were covered in the section 'Epidemiological features of SIDS infants'. The initial construction of this model thus first dealt with these epidemiological factors, after which the rest of the factors significant in the univariate analysis described in the section 'Univariate analysis of potentially modifiable risk factors' were added.

The results of first modelling the epidemiological characteristics significant in the univariate analysis are given in Table 3.56.

Highly significant factors included young mothers, larger families and infants with low birth weight for their gestation and sex. Both short gestation and admission to an SCBU were important factors. Receipt of Income Support, current unemployment and tenure of accommodation explained more of the variation between the two groups than other socio-economic deprivation markers such as weekly income, occupational status, poor education, overcrowding, lack of mobility or housing problems that especially affected the infant's room. The risk associated with males and multiple births just remained significant. Previous infant deaths and miscarriages did not remain significant, but previous stillbirths did. Marital status was not significant, but this is partially explained by the variable representing unwaged families which will include most of the single mothers. Other factors that were not significant included the time of antenatal booking, mothers who had an emergency caesarean section, infants with neonatal problems or congenital anomalies and infants resuscitated at delivery or given tube feeds.

Table 3.56 First stage empirical model: significant epidemiological features

Variable	Non-reference groups	OR (95% CI)	p-value
Maternal age	Continuous variable	2.19 (1.47–3.27)*	< 0.0001
Number of children (including index/control)	Two or three children	2.77 (1.81– 4.22)	< 0.0001
	Four or more	6.76 (3.44–13.26)	< 0.0001
Birth weight centiles	Continuous variable	1.41 (1.17–1.70)[†]	0.0003
Admission to SCBU	Infant admitted	2.58 (1.46–4.55)	0.0010
Income Support (IS)	Family received IS	2.20 (1.37–3.55)	0.0012
Gestational age	37–39 weeks	1.69 (1.17–2.43)	0.0049
	36 weeks or less	2.57 (1.31–5.04)	0.0059
No waged income	Parent(s) unemployed	1.78 (1.15–2.74)	0.0092
Housing tenure	Not owned or mortgage	1.72 (1.12–2.66)	0.014
Multiple births	Twins or triplets	3.95 (1.19–13.12)	0.025
Gender	Male	1.43 (1.01–2.01)	0.042
Previous stillbirth	At least one	3.59 (1.03–12.45)	0.044

Model includes 316 cases and 1 278 controls (98% of data). SCBU, special care baby unit

* OR based on 10-year intervals

[†] OR based on units of minus one standard deviation (i.e. risk is higher for smaller infants)

Epidemiological features that were significant in the univariate analysis but were not significant when added to the above model include: time of antenatal booking, delivery by caesarean section, neonatal problems, major congenital anomalies, treatments and procedures in the neonatal period, previous miscarriages, previous infant deaths, marital status, use of telephone, use of own transport, weekly income, occupational classification, parental education, housing problems that affected the infant's room and overcrowding

When the epidemiological variables with many missing values were added, paternal age, the council tax band of the accommodation and Apgar score at five minutes did not achieve significance, but the factors representing a short time between pregnancies and receipt of immunisation remained significant.

For over a third of all mothers, the most recent pregnancy was their first, so time between pregnancies was necessarily a 'missing' value for them. In order to include these mothers in the model, we dichotomised the interval between pregnancies with a cut-off at seven months and included all those for whom the pregnancy was their first in the group whose interval was greater than seven months (ie. the reference group). The effect of this would be to overestimate any difference between the two groups, as a larger proportion of control mothers had just one pregnancy compared to SIDS mothers, but when this alternative variable was added to the model it did not achieve significance (OR = 1.46 [95% CI: 0.83–2.56], p = 0.19).

For 5.4% of all infants, no information was available regarding immunisations. The univariate analysis shows that a greater proportion of control infants were immunised compared to the SIDS infants. When this factor was added to the above model, it remained significant and still remained significant when subsequent factors detailed below were added (OR = 0.25 [95% CI: 0.09–0.67]).

Table 3.57 shows the resultant model when the potentially modifiable risk factors significant in the univariate analysis are added. The factor representing infants being found with the head covered is the only factor related to events after the child was put down for the final or reference sleep. It is also the factor at this second stage with most missing values (2%). Two models are therefore represented in Table 3.57, the full empirical model including 'head covered' and the empirical model without this variable.

Entering variables purely on the basis of univariate significance rather than using a priori knowledge of the factors and relationships between them makes interpretation difficult. The difficulty lies in both the complex relationships between certain factors and, just as importantly, the lack of any relationship between other factors, which only serves to obscure what is already a complicated picture. The lack of stability in this over-fitted model is clearly demonstrated by the variability of the factors that appear in the resultant model at the 5% level when just one factor is removed. Reducing the arbitrary level of significance from the 5% level to the 1% level or lower does not eradicate the problem of interpretation but merely reduces the number of variables of interest. The final empirical model provides little in terms of definitive answers to our original hypotheses but is a good starting point for the multivariate analysis. The main purpose of the above model is to identify certain areas that require further investigation. These include:

- epidemiological characteristics and how they now relate to the risk factors;

- how the infant was positioned for sleep and eventually found;

- how the infant was covered;

- the items surrounding the infant in the sleeping place;

- where the infant slept in relation to the parents and potential adverse conditions that may affect the place of sleep;

- vulnerability of the infant at birth, during life and shortly before the last sleep;

- family disruption;

- exposure to tobacco smoke both during pregnancy and postnatally;

- relationship to pacifier use.

Using all the multivariate techniques previously described, together with the results from the univariate analyses, a summary and discussion of the findings for these areas is given in the next section.

Table 3.57 Second-stage empirical model: adding potentially modifiable risk factors

Variable	Non-reference group	Full empirical model		Excluding 'head covered'	
		OR (95% CI)	p-value	OR (95% CI)	p-value
Head covered	Yes	33.22 (9.46 to 116.69)	< 0.0001	–	–
Gestational age	37–39 weeks	1.74 (0.95 to 3.19)	0.07	1.49 (0.87 to 2.54)	0.14
	36 weeks or less	10.91 (3.90 to 30.50)	< 0.0001	2.71 (0.90 to 8.22)	0.08
Where infant slept*	Separate room	12.80 (5.00 to 32.76)	< 0.0001	7.25 (3.36 to 15.63)	< 0.0001
	Parent's bed	4.09 (1.84 to 9.11)	0.0006	3.01 (1.53 to 5.93)	0.0014
	Sofa with parent	53.85 (7.13 to 406.94)	< 0.0001	47.17 (3.77 to 590.94)	0.0028
Postnatal exposure to tobacco smoke	1–2 hours	1.89 (0.83 to 4.30)	0.13	1.05 (0.51 to 2.17)	0.90
	3–5 hours	1.41 (0.52 to 3.83)	0.50	1.53 (0.63 to 3.70)	0.35
	6–8 hours	7.03 (1.71 to 28.98)	0.007	4.37 (1.26 to 15.15)	0.02
	9 or more hours	12.37 (3.79 to 40.38)	< 0.0001	5.99 (2.12 to 16.93)	0.0007
Length of previous infant sleep	< 5 hours	1.89 (0.88 to 4.09)	0.10	2.62 (1.33 to 5.16)	0.0055
	> 10 hours	0.22 (0.09 to 0.52)	0.0007	0.22 (0.10 to 0.50)	0.0002
Sleep position	Put down on side	2.19 (1.23 to 3.91)	0.008	1.83 (1.07 to 3.13)	0.03
	Put down on front	6.78 (2.10 to 21.92)	0.0014	7.73 (2.70 to 22.12)	< 0.0001
Episodes of lifelessness	At least one	7.59 (2.14 to 26.93)	0.0017	4.68 (1.62 to 13.48)	0.0043
No waged income	Parent(s) unemployed	2.76 (1.45 to 5.25)	0.0019	2.17 (1.27 to 3.74)	0.005
Maternal alcohol consumption	>2 units in last 24 hours	7.83 (2.13 to 28.73)	0.0019	4.35 (1.54 to 13.22)	0.009
Maternal smoking	During pregnancy	2.58 (1.38 to 4.82)	0.0029	1.96 (1.14 to 3.36)	0.014
No. of children: (including index/controls)	Two or three	2.78 (1.45 to 5.34)	0.0022	3.08 (1.68 to 5.66)	0.0003
	Four or more	3.65 (1.36 to 9.82)	0.0103	5.98 (2.25 to 15.90)	0.0003
Moving house	Once in last year	1.73 (0.90 to 3.31)	0.1008	1.89 (1.05 to 3.41)	0.03
	Twice in last year	4.76 (1.30 to 17.47)	0.019	4.12 (1.34 to 12.65)	0.01
	Three or more times	8.93 (2.08 to 38.29)	0.0032	3.12 (0.86 to 11.34)	0.08
Used dummy	For last sleep	0.41 (0.22 to 0.77)	0.0056	0.47 (0.27 to 0.80)	0.006

Table 3.57 Second-stage empirical model: adding potentially modifiable risk factors, *cont.*

Variable	Non-ref group	Full empirical model		Excluding 'head covering'	
		OR (95% CI)	p-value	OR (95% CI)	p-value
Birth weight centiles	*Continuous variable*	1.55 (1.12 to 2.14)[†]	0.0077	1.08 (0.82 to 1.42)[†]	0.59
Infant health, last 24 hours	*Only fair*	2.33 (1.11 to 4.90)	0.026	1.27 (0.65 to 2.49)	0.49
	Poor	4.71 (1.24 to 17.91)	0.023	2.10 (0.48 to 9.23)	0.33
Pillow in cot	*For the last sleep*	5.72 (1.40 to 23.30)	0.015	4.09 (1.08 to 15.50)	0.039
Anxiety: thermal environment[‡]	*Too cold*	1.25 (0.60 to 2.60)	0.55	1.42 (0.73 to 2.77)	0.30
	Too hot	0.44 (0.23 to 0.87)	0.018	0.54 (0.30 to 0.97)	0.039
Feeding, last 24 hours	*Less than usual*	3.10 (1.09, 8.80)	0.033	1.40 (0.53 to 3.68)	0.50
Used a duvet	*For last sleep*	2.00 (1.03, 3.85)	0.039	1.60 (0.91 to 2.81)	0.10
Change in routine	*In last 24 hours*	2.35 (1.03, 5.36)	0.042	2.34 (1.10 to 4.95)	0.027
Maternal age	*Continuous variable*	1.78 (0.97, 3.26)[§]	0.061	2.32 (1.33 to 4.06)[§]	0.003
Paternal smoking	*Yes*	1.72 (0.96, 3.08)	0.066	2.05 (1.20 to 3.51)	0.009
Paternal drug abuse	*After birth*	3.28 (0.89, 12.04)	0.074	3.47 (1.15 to 10.50)	0.027
Baby Check score	*> 7*	1.58 [0.85, 2.93]	0.14	2.39 [1.44 to 3.96]	0.0007
Multiple births	*Twin or triplets*	4.08 (0.59, 28.39)	0.16	6.27 (1.27 to 30.88)	0.024
Admission to SCBU	*Yes*	1.46 (0.57, 3.74)	0.43	3.06 (1.49 to 6.26)	0.002

The shaded areas represent non-significant variables in one or other of the models or particular categories of a variable

Full empirical model includes 277 cases and 1 261 controls (95% of the data), second model includes 284 cases and 1 276 controls (96% of the data). SCBU, special care baby unit

* Reference group were those infants who shared a room with the parents, but not the parental bed

[†] OR based on units of one standard deviation

[‡] Reference group were those mothers not anxious about infant's thermal environment and those anxious about infant being too hot and cold

[§] OR based on 10-year intervals

Epidemiological variables significant in the first stage but not significant at this second stage include factors representing income support, housing tenure, gender and previous stillbirths

Risk factors that were significant in the univariate analysis but were not significant when added to the above model include: the mode of infant feeding and duration, maternal postnatal depression, other people smoking in the household, usual maternal alcohol consumption, usual and recent alcohol consumption of the partner, maternal use of illegal substances, the number of previous infant hospital admissions, infant health in the last week, infant medication in the last week. And for the last sleep: non-parental care, tog values of bedding and clothing when put down for the last sleep, whether the heating was on, whether the door was ajar, whether infant wore a hat, use of a cot bumper, whether the infant was sweating, how the bed covers were tucked in, softness of the mattress, the number of toys in the cot, use of listening devices

DISCUSSION

Data collection, case ascertainment and validity of the results

One of the priorities in the design of the CESDI SUDI study was to ensure that the data collected were as complete as possible, and that information was collected from both index and control families as soon as possible after the death of the index infants. The system for identifying the infants who had died was very effective; the study failed to identify only eight deaths of infants who should have been included during the three-year period. Data from public records (i.e. birth and death certificates) were thus obtained on 98.3% of eligible infants. The use of the families' own health visitors to make contact, together with the use of experienced health visitors and midwives to collect the data, resulted in a very high acceptance rate by the families, with virtually complete data sets being obtained from 93% of the SIDS and 92% of the non-SIDS families who were contacted. Regarding controls, the acceptance rate was also very high, with only 2.4% refusing to participate and replacement families being rapidly found for most of these, giving a final overall control data collection rate of 99.6%.

These ascertainment and enrolment figures are higher than for most previous similar studies and reduce the risk that the results are skewed by non-inclusion of an important minority group or groups [10-12].

Because of the detail of the information required about the precise circumstances of the deaths, it was important to ensure that this was collected as soon as possible after the event. The median time from the death of the index infant to notification to the CESDI researchers (14 hours), and from death until interview with the parents (four days) were both within the study design criteria (24 hours and five days, respectively), and demonstrate that, even in a large-scale population-based study of this nature, both rapid contact and high ascertainment and enrolment rates can be achieved. Indeed, it was the view of the researchers that the high enrolment rate was a direct consequence of the rapidity with which contact was made with both index and control families.

A further important feature of the study design was the age-matching of the control infants to the index infants. Because of the priority accorded to very rapid contact with index families, the delay in contacting the control families was slightly longer, although over 90% were interviewed within 12 days of the index infant's death. This longer delay meant that, by the time of the interview, the control infants were 11 days older than the index infants had been at death. This small age difference is unlikely to have had a major effect upon most of the factors being compared, especially for infants over two months of age (75% of the SIDS infants). For younger infants, however, and particularly for the factors reflecting patterns of infant care which were noted to change with age (e.g. bed-sharing, room-sharing, breast-feeding), this difference could be of importance and all statistical comparisons between the index and control infants were therefore adjusted to take account of age.

The study design used local health visitors to identify the control infants, as in previous studies in Avon [1,5]. We found that this ensured high levels of compliance. This design has been criticised on the basis that the geographical base for the practices of most health visitors would mean that the control infants were partially matched for locality of residence, and there would thus be a degree of inadvertent matching for socio-economic factors. Any inadvertent over-representation of the more socially deprived families amongst the controls would lead to an underestimate of the significance of any differences in social and economic factors found between index and control families.

In a previous study in Avon, we found that the use of control families identified randomly from the birth register led to a much higher rate of refusal to participate, and such refusals were more common amongst the more deprived groups, leading to a potential bias in the control population away from the more deprived groups. This led to the risk of *over*estimating the differences between index and control families [5,6,13]. The close similarities which we found when comparing the control families with families identified as having infants under one year of age in the UK 1991 Census for the South-West Region suggest that the control infants used in this study were representative of families with infants of this age.

This is the first large-scale study of SIDS in the UK after the 'Back to Sleep' campaign in 1991, and the largest population-based study of explained SUDI. Whilst it is not possible to be certain that the data from any study are completely free of systematic bias, the precautions taken in the design, conduct and analysis of the CESDI SUDI study have addressed such issues in detail, and allow the results to be interpreted with confidence. The close relationship which was established between the parents involved in the study and the research interviewers meant that sensitive and potentially painful information was readily given by the families. Information on paternity, drug and alcohol abuse was given by almost all families, in the knowledge that the information given was in strict confidence. An example of the trust established between the interviewers and the parents is the information given by the parents on parental occupation. Two families in the study gave the father's occupation as 'burglar'. This caused the researchers some difficulty in classification within the Registrar General's system, but the eventual consensus was that this constituted a semi-skilled manual occupation.

'Explained SUDI'

The findings paint an epidemiological profile for 'explained SUDI' that is similar in many respects to that seen in SIDS, both groups being at considerable social disadvantage. Common attributes include low birth weight and shorter gestation of the baby, younger maternal age but higher parity, poor educational attainment by parents, more unemployment, and lower socio-economic status and income.

The only epidemiological characteristics to differ with clear statistical significance between the 'explained SUDI' infants and those who died as SIDS were the distribution of age at death and parental smoking. The 'explained SUDI', like most other deaths in infancy, peaked in the first month, whilst SIDS peaked at three to four months of age. The incidence of smoking in pregnancy, whilst much higher amongst the mothers of 'explained SUDI' infants (49%) than the mothers of controls (27%), was even higher amongst the mothers of SIDS infants (66%). The significance of this comparison is further evidence that infant tobacco exposure is more than just an association with SIDS deaths. A greater proportion of the explained deaths included infants with congenital malformations at birth compared to SIDS infants, but as 14% of these deaths were due to congenital abnormality this comparison would be misleading.

Perhaps the most striking result was the finding that nearly half the babies showed signs of illness severe enough to need medical attention in the 24 hours before they died; the proportion would be greater if deaths from trauma were excluded from this analysis. This finding has important implications with regard to the education of parents and health professionals in the recognition of the severity of illness in babies. Some studies have shown that a proportion of explained sudden unexpected deaths of infants, particularly those related to infections or to trauma, may be preventable [1,14-17]. It is well known from the series of CESDI reports that failure to recognise severity of illness is a recurring theme, and that this failure of recognition may not only be by the parents but by health professionals who may give inappropriate reassurance that the baby is well.

Because of the heterogeneity of the deaths in this study the findings must be interpreted with caution. Although some overall differences between explained cases and controls have emerged, it is possible that distinctive characteristics of subgroups have been masked by dilution. The numbers in this study are not great enough to allow the subgroups to be analysed separately.

From the populations of the regions involved and from the periods of study in each, an approximate estimation can be made that each year throughout England and Wales about 120 infants may be dying in this category of 'explained SUDI'.

Epidemiology of SIDS

Many of the epidemiological features associated with SIDS found in previous studies have remained the same despite the fall in incidence. The majority of deaths occurred unobserved during the night-time sleep, and the same characteristic age distribution was still evident; very few deaths in the first month, a peak incidence at 12 weeks and a steady decline thereafter. SIDS was more prevalent in males and amongst multiple births, although neither factor was significant in the multivariate analysis. Vulnerability at birth was specifically represented in the models by short gestational age and low birth weight centiles. Male infants are heavier at birth, yet despite a predominance of males the SIDS infants in this study were of lower median birth weight, and despite controlling for short gestational age and maternal smoking during pregnancy the risk associated with infants born small remained significant. As well as being smaller for gestational age, SIDS infants had a higher chance of needing resuscitation at birth and of being admitted to a special care baby unit than control infants. Both young maternal age and high parity remained significant. Looking at the interaction of these two variables suggests that mothers of SIDS infants started having children at an earlier age and the number of subsequent births came at similar or shorter intervals than the infants born to the control mothers.

Some of these factors are clearly linked. Preterm babies and those born small for gestational age are inherently more likely to require significant resuscitation and be admitted to special care baby units. Furthermore, preterm delivery and poor intrauterine growth are not randomly distributed in the population, but share many of the social and economic antecedents that are known correlates with a risk of SIDS [18]. For this reason, the concept of a set of risk factors operating 'independently' is unhelpful, since there is more likely to be a set of causations linking adverse maternal factors to neonatal outcomes, which in turn contribute to the vulnerability of infants and increase their risk of SIDS. The concept of chains of causation, and the difficulties in analysis which may result, have been well described in the analogous problem of risk factors for neonatal encephalopathy [19].

Major epidemiological features which have changed since the reduction in incidence include a reduction in the previous high winter peaks of death and a shift of SIDS families to the more deprived social grouping. Previous studies found that the seasonal distribution was far more marked in infants aged over 12 weeks and an excess of male deaths in winter. However, in this study there was no difference in age distribution between infants who died in the colder months (October to March) or the warmer months (April to September). There was, however, a difference in gender, but in the opposite direction, a larger predominance of male deaths in the warmer months (70% SIDS males) rather than the cooler ones (58% SIDS males).

The excess of deaths amongst the infants in the most deprived social groups has been previously reported in studies dating from before as well as those which have followed risk reduction campaigns [5,10,12].

A striking feature of the present study, however, was the strong association of both explained and unexplained deaths with extreme poverty and socio-economic deprivation. Parents of index infants were younger, less well educated, had lower incomes, were more likely to be unemployed and, lived in less suitable housing which was commonly overcrowded. Mothers of index infants were less likely to have a supportive partner than were mothers of control infants. Many index families suffered the effects of multiple deprivation by these criteria. In the multivariate modelling process, indicators were used to represent socio-economic status, although none yielded a high enough correlation with other markers to be used as a sole proxy for deprivation. The most significant of these factors in this analysis was unemployment; nearly half the households of SIDS infants received no waged income.

A consistent thread through many of the cases was a background of social chaos often coupled with abject poverty. Indeed, the research interviewers encountered examples of poverty and deprivation of a degree which they could hardly believe was possible in late 20th-century Britain. This striking association of absolute poverty with the risk of infant death remains as clear as when first described by Templeman in 1892 [20].

In the past, it has been assumed that the infant risk factors (and many others) are specific to SIDS to the extent that the syndrome has been described as an 'epidemiological entity' [21]. However, in the univariate analysis, all of the infant characteristics significant amongst the SIDS group were similarly identified and tending in the same direction amongst the infants dying suddenly and unexpectedly from identified causes. Only the association with congenital malformations was significantly stronger for the non-SIDS deaths, whilst the association with maternal smoking was stronger for the SIDS infants. This observation suggests that, in general, sudden unexpected deaths in infancy share similar underlying factors, irrespective of the clinical or pathological findings, and this challenges a rigid concept of SIDS as an epidemiological entity.

Potentially modifiable risk factors

How the infant slept: prone, supine and side sleeping positions

Studies throughout the 1980s [5,13,22–31] consistently demonstrated an increased risk of SIDS for infants put down in the prone position. In seven of the 12 previous studies reporting this factor, including one study from the UK [5], within the *control* population prone sleeping was more prevalent than supine. The very low prevalence of prone sleeping position amongst control infants in the present study confirms the high uptake of the 'Back to Sleep' campaign message. Amongst the control infants, 67% usually slept supine at night, 30% were usually put down on their side and only 3% were usually put down prone. The risk associated with the prone position remains highly significant in all multivariate models, yet it is the least common position amongst SIDS infants.

The intervention campaign advising parents to avoid the prone position for infants appears to have been very successful, but some families have clearly not taken up this message. Given that the more deprived sections of the population are the least affected by public information campaigns, one might expect that the prevalence of prone sleeping position would be higher amongst the more deprived families. However, when the data are stratified for social class, the odds ratio for prone sleeping remains constant, and a smaller proportion of the more deprived SIDS families (social class V or unemployed) placed their infants prone (11%) compared to those in the other socio-economic groups (16%). The prevalence of prone sleeping position increases with increasing infant age, which suggests that parental practice is sometimes superseded by infant choice when the infant becomes old enough to change position. Very few SIDS infants found in the parental bed after the last sleep were put down prone

(2.5%), and relatively few (14.1%) found in the prone position as compared with SIDS infants who slept elsewhere (put down – 21.8%; found – 45.4%).

Part of the advice in 1991 was to use the side sleeping position as a safe alternative to the prone position. The results from the CESDI study confirm our previous observations [32] and those of others [10,11] that the side sleeping position, whilst less hazardous than the prone position, is associated with an increased risk when compared with the supine position, regardless of whether or not the infant's lower arm is extended to prevent rolling. Much (but not all) of the risk associated with the side position was related to the risk of the infant rolling into the prone position.

In the multivariate models, the odds ratio for side sleeping position was smaller than that for the prone position, but, because of the higher prevalence of side sleeping position, the population attributable risk (the number of deaths that would be prevented if the factor was eliminated) was higher for the side position (18.4%) compared to the prone position (14.2%). Further studies need to be conducted to establish the mechanism of risk for the side sleeping position, but it certainly should not be recommended as a safe alternative to sleeping supine.

Infant coverings, room heating and thermal environment

As in previous studies [5,33], SIDS infants in the present study were habitually more warmly wrapped than controls, and this difference persisted for the last/reference sleep. Both SIDS and control infants were substantially less heavily wrapped than in a previous study conducted in Avon [5] before the fall in the SIDS death rate, but the difference in thermal resistance of bedding between SIDS and controls was similar to that found previously (approximately 1 tog). Also similar to the Avon study was the observation that more SIDS than control infants slept in a room where the heating was on for the duration of the sleep.

In the multivariate analysis, the thermal resistance of the bedding and the room heating became non-significant, although maternal anxiety over infants becoming too hot remained in the model as an apparently protective factor, implying that this anxiety translated into a tendency for control mothers to keep their babies less warmly covered.

The effects of heavy wrapping on the infant's thermoregulatory ability is likely to be greater when infants sleep prone [34–36]. The absolute levels of thermal resistance used in the present study were much less than those in the earlier studies, which reflects the withdrawal in the early 1990s by manufacturers of the thick cot duvets (10–13 tog) previously widely used [5]. Thus, the apparently reduced effects of the thermal environment on the risk of SIDS in the present study is not unexpected.

In the present study, as in previous studies [1,37], being found with the head covered was a very strong risk factor in both univariate and multivariate analyses. Most of these infants were in cots, more than half had moved down under the covers and, as in the Dutch study [37], more than half were covered by infant duvets. Because the deaths are unobserved, one can only speculate as to whether head covering is part of a causal chain or a result of a struggle before death. For infants in cots, up to 80% of total heat loss may be from the head [6], and head covering may have a major effect upon thermoregulatory ability [34]. Because of the importance of the face as a site of heat loss when the infant is in bed, the use of bedding which can slip over the infant's head may have a major effect upon thermoregulation if the infant is supine. The study by Ponsonby [38] confirmed that for infants sleeping supine the use of a duvet was associated with a significantly increased risk of SIDS. L'Hoir postulated that a further part of the adverse effect of using a duvet may be an increased risk of the infant rolling from the side to the prone position [37]. Whatever the mechanism of the adverse effect of head covering, the risk associated with the use of bedding (notably duvets) which can slip over the baby's head is substantial. Advising parents to avoid duvets and tuck covers in firmly is an achievable aim and carries no identifiable danger to the infant.

The findings of this study support the 'Feet to Foot' campaign, launched in the UK by the Foundation for the Study of Infant Deaths, advising parents to place the feet of the infant at the foot of the cot, to avoid duvets and ensure that bedding is firmly tucked in.

What items surrounded the infant in the sleeping place?

Toys, cot bumpers, pillows and mattresses

A greater proportion of control infants had soft or hard toys and cot bumbers in the cot. None of these factors were significant when controlled for socio-economic status and maternal parity. However, the use of pillows in the cot either to prop the infant or use as a mattress was associated with a significantly increased risk in the multivariate analysis.

Whilst SIDS infants commonly slept on older mattresses than controls, this was accounted for by their lower socio-economic status and larger sibships. Amongst second or subsequent infants in a family, there was no difference in age of mattress between SIDS and control infants. This finding is in apparent conflict with the findings in Scotland by Brooke [12], in which use of a mattress that had been used before was identified as a risk factor, but in that study the age of the mattress was not ascertained. In neither study, however, was any evidence found to support the suggestion that fungal contamination of PVC-covered mattresses or toxic gas generation was a significant factor in the aetiology of SIDS [7].

For several infants, three of whom died, the parents had placed the infant to sleep on a pillow or other unsuitable bedding rather than a cot mattress because of parents' concerns about the risk of toxic gases from cot mattresses (see Chapter 5).

Pacifiers

There was no difference in the routine use of pacifiers ('dummies' or 'soothers') between SIDS and control infants, although there was a clear association between pacifier use and decreased prevalence and duration of breast-feeding. In both the univariate analysis and the multivariate models, it appeared that pacifier use on the last night/reference sleep was associated with a decreased risk of SIDS, a finding in agreement with those of previous investigators [37,39]. The reported adverse effects of pacifier use on breast-feeding rates [40], and the increased incidence of several markers of ill-health in infancy amongst regular pacifier users [41] suggest extreme caution in interpreting these results. The association between pacifier use and a reduced incidence of SIDS needs to be explored further because of the implications for infant care practices if evidence for a causal link should become strong. This will require knowledge of the physiological effects of pacifier use, awake and during sleep, in health and disease; further epidemiological studies to explore risk factors not captured in the existing studies; and a full evaluation of potential harm as well as potential benefit. No recommendations on pacifier use can be made in the light of the present knowledge.

Listening devices and 'apnoea' monitors

In the third year of the study, information was collected about the use of infant listening devices and apnoea monitors. The former were used by more control than SIDS families, although the apparent protective effect disappeared when account was taken of socio-economic status.

Apnœa monitors were used by 5% of SIDS infants and 2% of controls for the last/reference sleep.

This lack of any apparent value from such devices in the prevention of deaths is in agreement with previous studies [42]. If the control infants in this study are representative of infants in the UK, this would mean that home apnoea monitors are being used for around 14,000 infants in the UK each year. Given the lack of any good evidence of benefit to the infants from the use of such devices, the cost implications of providing this service need to be carefully addressed. For many families with infants who have experienced adverse events at home, and for those who have lost a previous infant suddenly and unexpectedly, the reassurance provided by the use of an apnoea monitor may justify its use, but suggesting to parents that the use of a monitor at home can be of medical benefit to infants deemed to be at increased risk (e.g. because of preterm birth) is not justified by our data or by previously published studies [43].

Where the infant slept

'Co-sleeping' is a term which encompasses a range of practices in which mothers and infants share the same environment for periods of sleep [44]. One form of co-sleeping, in which infants share the parental room rather than the bed, was the most common night-time sleeping practice amongst the control families and was associated with a decreased risk of SIDS. In the temporal model, the usual practice of bed-sharing (another form of co-sleeping) was not a significant factor, nor was bed-sharing for part of the last/reference sleep and then being put back in the cot. Bed-sharing for the whole of the last/reference sleep or being brought into the parental bed for the latter part of the sleep was associated with an increased risk of SIDS in the univariate analysis.

The apparent risk associated with bed-sharing increased in the empirical multivariate model. However, this type of model may not be appropriate because infants who shared their parent's bed were different in other important ways from those infants who slept in cots. For example, the prone position or covering of head by bedding were less frequent amongst bed-sharing than non-bed-sharing infants, so that inclusion of these risk factors in the multivariate model greatly increases the apparent risk associated with bed-sharing. If an a priori model is constructed incorporating factors relevant to bed-sharing such as recent maternal alcohol consumption, extreme overcrowding, parental lack of sleep and the use of duvets, the apparent risk of bed-sharing disappears. Furthermore, because of the high prevalence of parental smoking amongst the SIDS families in this study (84%), which was even higher amongst those parents found bed-sharing (91.5%), the risk associated with bed-sharing cannot be generalised to the whole population. From a birth population of approximately 500,000 only seven of the 321 (2.2%) SIDS infants for whom this information was available were found in the bed of non-smoking parents, compared to 103 of 1,299 (7.9%) control infants. Whilst not a protective factor, bed-sharing with non-smoking parents did not carry an increased risk of SIDS. This finding is in agreement with the data from a prospective study in New Zealand that followed a risk reduction campaign [11].

After controlling for other factors, there appears to be a highly increased independent risk of SIDS amongst infants who shared a sofa with a parent. Of the 20 SIDS infants (6.2 % of the total) found co-sleeping on a sofa the median age (nine weeks) was five weeks younger than those found elsewhere. Alcohol had been recently consumed by eight of the 20 parents which may have been a factor, but clearly this is in any case an inappropriate sleeping arrangement.

It is becoming clear from the published evidence that co-sleeping results in complex interactions between mothers and infants which are different to those found when mothers and infants sleep separately, and which need to be understood in detail before applying simplistic labels such as 'safe' or 'unsafe'. It appears from our analysis that it is not bed-sharing *per se* that is hazardous, but rather the particular circumstances in which bed-sharing may occur.

Vulnerability of the infant

As well as short gestation and low birth centiles, other factors suggesting vulnerability during life and shortly before death were identified in both univariate and multivariate analyses.

More SIDS than control infants were reported to have experienced one or more apparent life-threatening events. The recall of these events may have been subject to bias, as SIDS parents may have interpreted previous minor episodes as more important than they actually were. However, of those reporting such episodes, a similar proportion of SIDS and control infants had experienced more than one, or had called the general practitioner or taken the infant to hospital, which suggests that this bias was limited. This factor remained significant in both empirical multivariate models, but since the episodes were of varied and unknown cause, it is not possible to define the type that was associated with an increased risk of subsequent SIDS. Similarly, as noted above, we found no evidence that the use of apnoea monitors or other monitoring devices was of value in preventing deaths.

In the 24 hours before death, significantly more SIDS parents than controls thought the health of their infant was poor and feeding was less than normal. These findings are similar to those noted above for the 'explained SUDI' (see the section 'Explained SUDI' above). According to the Baby Check score, over a fifth of SIDS infants were unwell in the 24 hours preceding death, a higher proportion than in the previous Avon study [9] or the New Zealand study [45], both of which preceded SIDS risk reduction campaigns. The majority of the SIDS infants, especially the younger ones, displayed minor signs or symptoms. For the small proportion of infants showing signs of being severely unwell, appropriate action by parents or healthcare professionals might have prevented death. Although over three-quarters of SIDS infants appeared healthy just before the last sleep, these findings suggest that not all SIDS infants were healthy and normal. If Baby Check had been widely used, some of the SIDS infants would have been under medical observation at the time at which they died, although whether this would have changed the outcome is speculative. Clearly, there is a need for more detailed evaluation of the use of Baby Check as part of routine infant surveillance.

Events described by parents which have been found to be significant in other studies include cyanotic attacks [24] and convulsions [46]. Several studies have looked at signs of illness preceding death and found specific symptoms amongst SIDS infants, including respiratory problems, irritability, rash, change of cry, fever, [47] gastro-intestinal illness [18,23,24,46] and maternal reports of infants becoming sleepy, listless and droopy [18,47]. Collectively, minor signs of illness before death appear to be more prevalent amongst SIDS infants, although there appears to be no difference in major signs of illness [48] or unreported severe illness [14,49]. The potential for preventing some SIDS by recognition of illness remains controversial [49]. Many of the antecedent factors noted in our study could be ascertained objectively from existing medical records, but none were sufficiently specific to allow any particular individual intervention to be targeted at those infants most at risk of SIDS.

In contrast, the Baby Check score is a means of quantifying actual illness, can be used by parents as a guide to the advisability and urgency of seeking medical attention, and can be used by health professionals as a triage tool to discriminate more reliably between those infants who should be assessed in hospital and those who need no such assessment [3]. It focuses attention on infants who are potentially ill as opposed to those who might become ill, and therefore has the possible capability to trigger interventions which could be life-saving.

Retroprospective scoring of the Baby Check leaves open the possibility of recall bias, and limitation of the maximum score to 96 might lead to an underestimation of the severity of illness. Parental recognition of fever was used as a proxy for a temperature measurement. Recent work [50] suggests that touch usually identifies the presence of a fever but may overestimate it. On this dimension, the score may overestimate the severity of illness for some infants. However, the similarity of results obtained when we exclude this symptom from the composite score suggest the effect is minimal

The SUDI confidential enquiries have repeatedly identified failure to recognise the severity of illness, sometimes by the parents but often by healthcare professionals. While there are clear general messages for the necessity of better professional education and training, the use of the Baby Check score evidently has the potential to guide less confident or experienced workers in their decisions. The evidence from the explained deaths suggests an even greater potential for prevention of these deaths.

We were concerned at the level of discordance between the Baby Check score and the parental recognition of ill health in their baby, which occurred quite commonly in the control group as well as in the SIDS families. Some parents find it difficult to communicate their concerns about their baby's health, and the use of the Baby Check may help them to assess or describe illness more accurately. A further benefit of the Baby Check may be that, by enabling parents to recognise when illness may be serious, it reduces the frequency of inappropriate demands on the primary care team.

Immunisations

Despite a complete lack of good evidence, the media have raised public concern that routine childhood immunisations may increase the risk of SIDS. In the present study, we confirmed the findings from New Zealand [51] that immunisation was associated with a significantly *lower* risk of SIDS, and this finding was independent of infant age, socio-economic status and maternal smoking. The fall in the incidence of SIDS in the UK has occurred over a period during which the uptake of infant immunisations has increased, and it followed closely the change in 1990 of the timing of the first immunisation from three months to two months of age. There is thus good evidence, both demographic and epidemiological, that immunisation in infancy is associated with a reduction of the risk of SIDS, and parents should be reassured accordingly.

Family disruption

As well as social deprivation, which was represented in the multivariate analysis by unemployment, social disruption in terms of families moving accommodation also remained significant. The risk associated with moving house increased with the number of moves of accommodation. In the temporal model, moving house before the birth remained significant, but moving house after the infant was born did not. This suggests that moving home may be a marker of insecurity of tenure and consequent lack of a stable support network rather than a marker of acute disruption near to the time of the infant's death. Recent major changes in normal routine (e.g. going on holiday or visiting friends or relatives) were also more common in SIDS families than in controls. These findings are in general agreement with those of Ford [52], in New Zealand, who found an increased incidence of significant life events amongst SIDS families.

The concerns raised over the risks of SIDS posed by young infants making long airline flights [53] were not substantiated in this study, none of the infants who died ever having been on an aeroplane. By extrapolation from the controls in this study, we estimate that around 2,400 English infants travel on long haul flights each year. Thus, any increase in risk must be very small [54].

Social deprivation and disruption have strong associations with drug abuse, alcohol consumption and parental smoking. In the multivariate analyses, controlling for unemployment and moving accommodation, some of these associations disappear. However, maternal alcohol consumption in the 24 hours before the last/reference sleep and various factors representing parental smoking remained significant. Recent alcohol consumption may be a contributory factor to the risk associated with bed-sharing, as discussed above.

The increasing proportion of mothers who return to work soon after the birth of their infants led to concerns that care of such infants by child-minders or babysitters might increase the risk of SIDS, as studies in the US have shown that child-minders may be less well informed about ways of reducing the risk of SIDS [55]. In the present study, whilst significantly more of the SIDS than control infants were looked after by babysitters in the 24 hours before the last/reference sleep, no infants died whilst under the supervision of a child-minder or babysitter.

Anecdotal reports of infants dying after being left unchecked for long periods of time led to the question of whether SIDS infants had been checked more or less frequently during the last sleep compared with control infants during the reference sleep. Whilst SIDS infants were discovered dead, on average, one hour later than the time the control infants awoke from the reference sleep, this was not because they had been left for a longer period. They had in fact been put to bed considerably later than the control infants, and had been left for a significantly *shorter* period. This pattern of going to bed later and getting up later was characteristic of the families of SIDS infants and may in part be related to their very high unemployment rates. A further important difference in the sleeping patterns of SIDS and control infants became apparent in considering the longest sleeps which the infants had experienced in the 24 hours before the beginning of the last/reference sleep. During this period, the longest uninterrupted sleep period for the SIDS infants was significantly shorter than for the control infants. Indeed, a reported sleep period of more than 10 hours was associated with a significantly reduced risk of SIDS. Since around three-quarters of both SIDS and control parents thought that this sleep duration was typical for their infant, it would seem that in general SIDS infants sleep for shorter periods than do control infants. Whether this is an innate characteristic of the infants, or is related to the differing life styles of the SIDS and control families is not clear, although it is clear from the parents' responses that short sleep periods for the infants are accompanied by an interrupted sleep pattern for the parents. An anticipated concomitant of this observation would be that more of the SIDS parents than the parents of control infants would have been very tired at the time of the last/reference sleep. The effect that such tiredness might have upon parents' ability to respond to their infant during periods when parents are asleep is not clear, but arousal thresholds for the parents might be expected to be higher in such circumstances. Bed-sharing with an infant for whom the maximum period of sleep in the preceding 24 hours was four hours or less was shown in the multivariate analysis to be associated with an increased risk of SIDS (see above). Such an effect supports the suggestion that sleep deprivation in the carer may have potential adverse effects under such circumstances, although the mechanism remains obscure.

A further factor which might adversely affect the ability of mothers to respond appropriately to their infants is postnatal depression, which has been shown to be associated with an increased risk of SIDS [56].

Our study was not primarily aimed towards quantifying postnatal depression, and the data set was limited to maternal self-report and professionals' records, which cannot be validated and which are highly susceptible to bias. The self-reported rates were twice as high as those reported by professionals, so it is possible that, whilst mothers were prepared to admit depressive symptoms to the research interviewer (as a neutral person), they may have feared the consequences of such an admission to other professionals. Overall, about a fifth of the mothers of SIDS infants and a sixth of the controls admitted to depressive symptoms. Severe depression, although uncommon, was found significantly more frequently amongst the mothers of SIDS than control infants.

A possible increase in the risk of SIDS is not the only consequence of postnatal depression. There are well documented effects upon infant development [57], and these may cast a shadow much further into childhood. Since postnatal depression is a treatable condition, recognition of depression and the provision of appropriate help for depressed mothers remains an important public health issue.

Postnatal depression can, in principle, be quantified with reasonable precision using the Edinburgh Postnatal depression scale [58]. However, there is some evidence that anxious mothers may also score highly on the scale [59], which would considerably reduce its specificity. Furthermore its use after an infant has died as SIDS cannot be an accurate assessment of its value before the death. Mitchell and colleagues [56] prospectively collected population-based data on postnatal depression and were able to show a nearly threefold difference in incidence between those mothers who subsequently lost a baby as SIDS and control mothers. They also enquired about psychiatric illness in general in the New Zealand case-control study and found a significant association between the risk of SIDS and maternal use of psychotropic medication, maternal admission to hospital for psychiatric illness and family history of postnatal depression.

The factors increasing the risk of clinical depression following childbirth are very similar to the factors associated with an increased risk of SIDS. The question, therefore, is whether the existence of depression in the mother is an independent factor adding to the pre-existing risk of SIDS, or whether it is merely a marker for adverse events in the prenatal, intrapartum or postnatal period which are themselves the factors predisposing to SIDS. Unfortunately, neither the results of our study nor those of Mitchell disentangles the issue of whether postnatal depression (or other maternal psychiatric illness) is an independent factor. Further carefully designed and controlled studies will need to be undertaken if this issue is to be adequately resolved.

Breast-feeding

In this study, as in a previous study in the UK [60], we found a significant protective effect from breast-feeding in the univariate analysis, but no evidence of a dose-response effect – the apparent protection from breast-feeding for just one week was virtually identical to that from prolonged exclusive breast-feeding. These results suggest that the protection observed may be more a marker of the life style of the families in which mothers chose to breast-feed rather than a direct benefit from breast-feeding. The prevalence of breast-feeding was much higher amongst the more affluent families and was inversely related to the prevalence of maternal smoking. In the multivariate model the effects of breast-feeding ceased to be significant once maternal smoking or socio-economic status were included in the model. These findings are very similar to previous Avon data from before the 'Back to Sleep' campaign in the UK [60], and to the prospective study which followed the risk reduction campaign in New Zealand [11]. Breast-feeding has many important advantages to the infant, in terms of protection from infection, growth and possibly developmental progress, but it does not have a direct protective effect against the risk of SIDS.

Exposure to tobacco smoke

More than 20 studies conducted before the fall in SIDS rate have investigated maternal smoking during pregnancy and nearly all found a significant association [61]. More recent studies in New Zealand [11], Sweden [10], Norway [62] and preliminary analysis from the first two years of this study [63] suggest the association is now stronger and independent of other risk factors. Results from the whole three-year data set confirm the interim findings and suggest a further risk from postnatal exposure of tobacco smoke. Maternal smoking during pregnancy demonstrated a strong dose-response effect in the univariate analysis, the risk increasing with increasing cigarette consumption by the mother. When the data were stratified for socio-economic status, the prevalence of smoking for all mothers in this study was higher amongst the more deprived groups, but the difference between the SIDS and control mothers remained constant across all social strata. In the multivariate analysis, both maternal smoking during pregnancy and postnatal exposure remained significant and independent of each other. Postnatal exposure could be represented by paternal smoking or a parental estimation of the infant's daily exposure, which showed a clear biological gradient; the more hours the infant was exposed to smoke the greater the risk.

In only 16% of SIDS households did neither parent smoke. The population-attributable risk for smoking by at least one parent was 61%.

Smoking in pregnancy retards fetal growth and neurological development [64–66] and a correlation between this exposure and brainstem gliosis associated with hypoxic-ischaemic events has recently been found in SIDS infants [67]. It is difficult to separate completely the effects of *in utero* exposure from those of exposure in infancy, as most mothers who smoke in pregnancy continue to do so after the birth of their infants. Exposure *in utero* from smokers other than the mother is likely to result in the fetus receiving a lower dose of the various toxins than if the mother smokes. Our data, which show a very strong dose-response association between the risk of SIDS and the daily smoke exposure in infancy, support the suggestion that both prenatal and postnatal exposure to tobacco smoke have effects on the risk of SIDS. This is further supported by the results of our multivariate analysis, in which smoke exposure before and after birth remain as separate and apparently independent adverse effects.

In the absence of experimental evidence, regarded by many as a necessary and sufficient condition for identifying causal associations, a number of criteria have been identified which, taken together, would make it 'more provident to act on the basis that the association is causal rather than to await further evidence' [61]. These criteria are based on those set out by Bradford Hill [68] and include strength and consistency of findings between studies, biological plausibility, coherence with other known facts and, where applicable, a temporal sequence and biological gradient. Certainly, the first two of these criteria have been fulfilled. The evidence from previous studies consistently supported a strong association between SIDS and maternal smoking during pregnancy [61]. Evidence from the present study, after the 'Back to Sleep' campaign and the subsequent fall in incidence of SIDS in the UK continues to show a strong relationship between maternal smoking and the risk of SIDS. Similar results have recently been reported from the Nordic countries [62,69] and from New Zealand [11] after risk reduction campaigns for SIDS in those countries. The findings were both consistent over different socio-economic strata, and despite the high prevalence of maternal smoking amongst the explained deaths, the proportion of smokers amongst SIDS mothers was significantly higher. Clearly, the association of smoking with the risk of SIDS is biologically plausible. The criterion for a temporal sequence has also been fulfilled, as the risk factor precedes the event, in this case death. Finally, a biological gradient has clearly been demonstrated, with the dose-response effect both during pregnancy and with postnatal exposure.

It thus appears that, despite the absence of direct experimental evidence, the relationship between smoking and SIDS is probably causal. Measures to reduce the exposure of infants to tobacco smoke, both before and after birth, should therefore be viewed as a priority. The lack of success of previous programmes aimed at stopping women from smoking in pregnancy should not deter further attempts to achieve this end, but 'harm reduction' approaches which aim at reducing rather than preventing smoking may be more successful. The institution of 'smoke free zones' in the homes of infants may be more acceptable to families in which smoking occurs, and the data from the CESDI study on the steepness of the dose-response curve for postnatal exposure to tobacco smoke may facilitate the acceptance of this concept. As previously suggested [63], minimising the exposure of infants to tobacco smoke is the responsibility of all smokers. Smoking in the presence of pregnant women or young infants should be viewed as being as unacceptable as drinking and driving.

Alcohol and illicit drug use

Whilst regular moderate or heavy alcohol intake (more than 10 units per week), and particularly 'binge' drinking, by mothers during pregnancy and the postnatal period was associated with a significantly increased risk of SIDS, no such effects were seen for mothers who consumed between one and 10 units per week. Indeed, there was a slightly lower risk of SIDS for infants of mothers who consumed between one and 10 units per week when compared with those who consumed no alcohol at all. This should not be interpreted as a protective effect of alcohol, as total abstinence from alcohol may be associated with other potentially adverse behavioural patterns in a society in which some alcohol intake is the usual pattern. However, these observations are compatible with the 'J shaped curve' seen for adverse health effects of alcohol in adults. Clearly, given the well-known adverse effect upon the fetus of moderate alcohol intake, our data do not suggest that alcohol intake in pregnancy is safe. More detailed studies are required before recommendations can be made about 'safe' levels of alcohol intake for women with young children.

Alcohol intake above two units by mothers in the 24 hours before the last/reference sleep was, however, associated with a highly significant increase in the risk of SIDS, particularly for mothers sharing a bed (or sofa) with their infant. This finding remained highly significant in all multivariate models.

Abstinence or heavy drinking by partners was also associated with a higher risk of SIDS, although this was less significant than for the mothers, perhaps because partners were not involved in infant care.

A significantly higher proportion of SIDS than control mothers admitted to using illegal substances on more than one occasion before, during and after pregnancy. A surprising finding was that 2.6% of the control mothers were habitual users of illegal substances after their baby had been born. The proportions of regular users during and after the pregnancy were higher amongst SIDS partners (14.8%) than amongst the controls (4.5%), and this difference remained significant in some but not all multivariate models. The drug most commonly used by all groups was cannabis. Because almost all cannabis users also smoked tobacco, it was not possible to identify a separate risk from cannabis use.

Infants and families at risk

Overall, in the population included in this study the SIDS rate was 0.768 per 1,000 live births, i.e. approximately one baby in 1,300 died as SIDS. From our data, it is possible to identify within the population a number of factors which are associated with an increased risk of SIDS. The identification of families at higher risk of SIDS is of importance in allowing the appropriate deployment of scarce health care resources, and in attempting to achieve changes in life style or patterns of child care that might reduce this risk. For families already at low risk, knowledge of the factors influencing risk may help to provide reassurance and encouragement in continuing appropriate patterns of care.

Table 3.58 shows the three prenatal factors with the highest predictive value (based on the Wald Score) of an increased risk of SIDS, and the likely effect of the presence or absence of each factor on the incidence of SIDS, along with the effect when combining these factors.

Thus, an infant living in a household in which nobody smoked had a risk of SIDS of around one in 5,000, whilst if anyone in the household smoked this risk rose to around one in 700. Similarly for an infant in a household in which there was no waged income, the risk was around one in 500, compared with one in 2,000 if there was a waged income.

Table 3.58 SIDS rates for different factors based on the data from the CESDI SUDI study

	SIDS rate per 1000 live births*	SIDS incidence in this group*
Overall rate in the study population	0.768	1 in 1 303
Rate for groups with different factors		
Anybody smokes in the household	1.357	1 in 737
Nobody smokes in the household	0.199	1 in 5 041
No waged income in household	2.057	1 in 486
At least one waged income in household	0.479	1 in 2 088
Mother < 27 years and parity >1	1.762	1 in 567
Mother > 26 years or parity = 1	0.531	1 in 1 882
None of these factors	0.117	1 in 8 543
One of these factors	0.619	1 in 1 616
Two of these factors	1.678	1 in 596
All three of these factors	4.674	1 in 214

* Based on the number of live births in each study region from 1993 to 1995 inclusive (OPCS)

The correlation between the factors was taken into account when more than one factor was used to calculate the rate, but because all three factors are independently significant in the multivariate analyses, the presence of more than one will have an increased effect.

Thus, it can be seen that for infants in families in which all three factors are present the risk of SIDS was one in 214, compared with a risk of one in 8,543 for infants in families with none of the factors, i.e. a 40-fold difference in risk.

Since the factors will generally remain the same (with the possible exception of maternal age below 27 years), the risk of SIDS to a subsequent child in a family in which one infant has already died will range from one in 214 to one in 8,543. This does not take account of possible familial incidence of factors other than those included in Table 3.58.

For a family with none of these three factors, the risk of two infants dying as SIDS by chance alone will thus be one in (8,543 × 8,543), i.e. approximately one in 73 million. For a family with all three factors, the risk will be one in (214 × 214), i.e. approximately one in 46,000. Thus, for families with several known risk factors for SIDS, a second SIDS death, whilst uncommon, is 1,600 times more likely than for families with no such factors. Where additional adverse factors are present, the recurrence risk would correspondingly be greater still.

Whilst child abuse and non-accidental injury are associated with many of the same factors as an increased risk of SIDS (see Chapter 5), the increased risk in the above calculation is derived from a population in which careful attempts have been made to exclude those deaths for which abuse by a parent or carer was identified as a probable causal factor. When a second SIDS death occurs in the same family, in addition to a careful search for an inherited disorder there must always be a very thorough investigation of the circumstances – although it would be inappropriate to assume maltreatment was always the cause.

References

1. Gilbert, R, Rudd, P, Berry, PJ, Fleming, PJ, Hall, E, White, DG, Oreffo, VO, James, P and Evans, JA. 'Combined effect of infection and heavy wrapping on the risk of sudden unexpected infant death', *Archives of Disease in Childhood*, 1992; 67(2): 171–7.

2. Rognum, TO and Willinger, M. 'The story of the Stavanger definition' in Rognum, TO (ed.) *Sudden Infant Death Syndrome: New Trends in the Nineties*. Oslo: Scandinavian University Press, 1995: 21–5.

3. Morley, CJ, Thornton, AJ, Cole, TJ, Hewson, PH and Fowler, MA. 'Baby Check: a scoring system to grade the severity of acute illness in babies under 6 months old', *Archives of Disease in Childhood*, 1991; 66: 100–106.

4. Cole, TJ. 'Conditional reference charts to assess weight gain in British infants', *Archives of Disease in Childhood*, 1995; 73: 8–16.

5. Fleming, PJ, Gilbert, R, Azaz, Y, Berry, PJ, Rudd, PT, Stewart, A and Hall, E. 'Interaction between bedding and sleeping position in the sudden infant death syndrome: a population based case-control study', *British Medical Journal*, 1990; 301(6743): 85–9.

6. Wigfield, RE, Fleming, PJ, Azaz, YEZ, Howell, TE, Jacobs, DE, Nadin, PS, McCall, MJ and Stewart, AJ. 'How much wrapping do babies need at night?', *Archives of Disease in Childhood*, 1993; 69: 181–6.

7. Limerick, S (chair). *The Report of the Expert Group to Investigate Cot Death Theories: Toxic Gas Hypothesis*. London: Department of Health, 1998.

8. Kemp, JS, Livne, M, White, DK and Arfken, CL. 'Softness and potential to cause rebreathing: differences in bedding used by infants at high and low risk for sudden infant death syndrome', *Journal of Pediatrics*, 1998; 132(2): 234–9.

9. Cole, TJ, Gilbert, RE, Fleming, PJ, Morley, CJ, Rudd, PT and Berry, PJ. 'Baby Check and the Avon infant mortality study', *Archives of Disease in Childhood*, 1991; 66(9): 1077–8.

10. Oyen, N, Markestad, T, Skjaerven, R, Irgens, LM, Helweg-Larsen, K, Alm, B, Norvenius, G and Wennergren, G. 'Combined effects of sleeping position and prenatal risk factors in sudden infant death syndrome: the Nordic epidemiological SIDS study', *Pediatrics*, 1997; 100(4): 613–21.

11. Mitchell, EA, Tuohy, PG, Brunt, JM, Thompson, JMD, Clements, MS, Stewart, AW, Ford, RPK and Taylor, BJ. 'Risk factors for sudden infant death syndrome following the prevention campaign in New Zealand: a prospective study', *Pediatrics*, 1997; 100(5): 835–40.

12. Brooke, H, Gibson, A, Tappin, D and Brown, H. 'Case-control study of sudden infant death syndrome in Scotland 1992–5', *British Medical Journal*, 1997; 314: 1516–20.

13. Wigfield, RE, Fleming, PJ, Berry, PJ, Rudd, PT and Golding J. 'Can the fall in Avon's sudden infant death rate be explained by changes in sleeping position?', *British Medical Journal*, 1992; 304: 282–3.

14. Clarke, J, Davidson, MM, Downham, MAPS, Ferris JAJ *et al.* 'Newcastle survey of deaths in early childhood 1974/76, with special reference to sudden unexpected deaths', *Archives of Disease in Childhood*, 1977; 528: 28–35.

15. Knowelden, J, Keeling, J and Nicholl, JP. *A multicentre study of post-neonatal mortality*. Crown Copyright, 1984.

16. Moore, A. 'Preventable childhood deaths in Wolverhampton', *British Medical Journal*, 1986; 293: 656–8.

17. Taylor, EM and Emery, JL. 'Family and community factors associated with infant deaths that might be preventable', *British Medical Journal*, 1983; 287: 871–4.

18. Hoffman, HJ and Hillman, IS. 'Epidemiology of the Sudden Infant Death Syndrome: maternal, neonatal and postneonatal risk factors', *Clinical Perinatology*, 1992; 19: 717–37.

19. Badawi, N, Kurinczuk, JJ, Keogh, JM *et al.* 'Antepartum risk factors for newborn encephalopathy: the Western Australia case control study', *British Medical Journal*, 1999; 317: 549–53.

20. Templeman, C. 'Two hundred and fifty-eight cases of suffocation in infants', *Edinburgh Medical Journal*, 1892; 38: 322–9.

21. Daltveit, AK, Oyen, N, Skjaerven, R and Irgens, LM. 'The epidemic of SIDS in Norway 1967–93: changing effects of risk factors', *Archives of Disease in Childhood*, 1997; 77: 23–7.

22. Tonkin, SL. 'Epidemiology of cot deaths in Auckland', *New Zealand Medical Journal*, 1986; 99(801): 324–6.

23. Kahn, A, Blum, D, Hennart, P, Sellens, C, Samson-Dollfus, D, Tayot, J, Gilly, R, Dutruge, J, Flores, R and Sternberg, B. 'A critical comparison of the history of sudden-death infants and infants hospitalised for near-miss for SIDS', *European Journal of Pediatrics*, 1984; 143(2): 103–7.

24. Cameron, MH and Williams, AL. 'Development and testing of scoring systems for predicting infants with high-risk of sudden infant death syndrome in Melbourne', *Australian Paediatric Journal*, 1986; 22 (supplement 1): 37–45.

25. de Jonge, GA, Engelberts, AC, Koomen-Liefting, AJM and Kostense, PJ. 'Cot death and prone sleeping position in the Netherlands', *British Medical Journal*, 1989; 298: 722.

26. McGlashann, ND. 'Sudden infant deaths in Tasmania, 1980–1986: a seven-year prospective study', *Social Science and Medicine*, 1989; 29(8): 1015–26.

27. Lee, NNY, Chan, YF, Davis, DP, Lau, E and Yip, DCP. 'Sudden infant death syndrome in Hong Kong: confirmation of a low incidence', *British Medical Journal*, 1989; 298: 721.

28. Mitchell, EA, Ford, RP, Taylor, BJ, Stewart, AW, Becroft, DM, Scragg, R, Barry, DM, Allen, EM, Roberts, AP and Hassall, IB. 'Further evidence supporting a causal relationship between prone sleeping position and SIDS', *Journal of Paediatrics and Child Health*, 1992; 28 (supplement 1): S9–S12.

29. Ponsonby, AL, Dwyer, T, Gibbons, LE, Cochrane, JA and Wang, YG. 'Factors potentiating the risk of sudden infant death syndrome associated with the prone position', *New England Journal of Medicine*, 1993; 329(6): 377–82.

30. Dwyer, T, Ponsonby, AL, Newman, NM and Gibbons, LE. 'Prospective cohort study of prone sleeping position and sudden infant death syndrome', *Lancet*, 1991; 337(8752): 1244–7.

31. Klonoff-Cohen, HS and Edelstein, SL. 'A case-control study of routine and death scene sleep position and sudden infant death syndrome in Southern California', *JAMA*, 1995; 273(10): 790–4.

32. Fleming, PJ, Blair, PS, Bacon, C, Bensley, D, Smith, I, Taylor, E, Berry, J, Golding, J and Tripp, J. 'Environment of infants during sleep and risk of sudden infant death syndrome: results of 1993–5 case-control study for confidential enquiry into stillbirths and deaths in infancy', *British Medical Journal*, 1996; 313: 191–8.

33. Ponsonby, AL, Dwyer, T, Gibbons, LE, Cochrane, JA, Jones, ME and McCall, MJ. 'Thermal environment and sudden infant death syndrome: case-control study', *British Medical Journal*, 1992; 304(6822): 277–82.

34. Sawczenko, A and Fleming, PJ. 'Thermal Stress, Sleeping Position, and the Sudden Infant Death Syndrome', *Sleep*, 1996; 19(10): S267–S270.

35. Tuffnell, CS, Petersen, SA and Wailoo, MP. 'Prone sleeping infants have a reduced ability to lose heat', *Early Human Development*, 1995; 43: 2109–116.

36. Skadberg, B and Markestad, T. 'Behaviour and physiological responses during prone and supine sleep in early infancy', *Archives of Disease in Childhood*, 1997; 763: 20–4.

37. L'Hoir, MP, Engelberts, AC, van Well, GThJ, McClelland, S, Westers, P, Dandachli, T, Mellenbergh, GJ, Wolters, WHG and Uber, J. 'Risk and preventative factors for cot death in the Netherlands, a low-incidence country', *European Journal of Pediatrics*, 1998; 157: 681–8.

38. Ponsonby, AL, Dwyer,T, Couper, D and Cochrane, J. 'Association between the use of a quilt and Sudden Infant Death Syndrome: case-control study', *British Medical Journal*, 1998; 316: 195–6.

39. Mitchell, EA, Taylor, BJ, Ford, RP, Stewart, AW, Becroft, DM, Thompson, JM, Scragg, R, Hassall, IB, Barry, DM and Allen, EM. 'Dummies and the sudden infant death syndrome', *Archives of Disease in Childhood*, 1993; 68(4): 501–4.

40. Victora, CG, Behague, DP, Barros, FC, Olinto, MTA and Weiderpass, E. 'Pacifier use and short breastfeeding duration: cause, consequence, or coincidence?', *Pediatrics*, 1997; 99: 445–53.

41. North, K, Fleming, PJ, Golding, J and the ALSPAC study team. 'Pacifier Use and Morbidity in

the First Six Months of Life', *Pediatrics Electronic Pages*, 1999; 103(3): e34.

42. Ward, SL, Keens, TG, Chan, LS, Chipps, BE *et al.* 'Sudden Infant Death Syndrome in infants evaluated by apnea programmes in California', *Pediatrics*, 1986; 77: 451–5.

43. Hodgman, JE. 'Apnea of Prematurity and Risk for SIDS', *Pediatrics*, 1998; 102(4): 969–71.

44. McKenna, J, Mosko, SS and Richard, CA. 'Bedsharing promotes breastfeeding', *Pediatrics*, 1997; 100(2): 214–19.

45. Taylor, BJ, Williams, SM, Mitchell, EA and Ford, RP. 'Symptoms, sweating and reactivity of infants who die of SIDS compared with community controls', *Journal of Paediatrics and Child Health*, 1996; 32(4): 316–22.

46. Rintahaka, PJ and Hirvonen, J. 'The epidemiology of sudden infant death syndrome in Finland in 1969–1980', *Forensic Science International*, 1986; 30(2–3): 219–33.

47. Carpenter, RG, Gardner, A, Pursall, E, McWeeny, PM and Emery, JL. 'Identification of some infants at immediate risk of dying unexpectedly and justifying intensive study', *Lancet*, 1979; 2(8138): 343–6.

48. Gilbert, RE, Fleming, PJ, Azaz, Y and Rudd, PT. 'Signs of illness preceding sudden unexpected death in infants', *British Medical Journal*, 1990; 300(6734): 1237–9. [Erratum appears in *BMJ*, 1990; 300(6736): 1378.]

49. Ford, RP, Mitchell, EA, Stewart, AW, Scragg, R and Taylor, BJ. 'SIDS, illness, and acute medical care', *Archives of Disease in Childhood*, 1997; 77(1): 54–5.

50. Whybrew, K, Murray, M and Morley, C. 'Diagnosing fever by touch: observational study', *British Medical Journal*, 1998; 317: 321.

51. Mitchell, EA, Stewart, AW and Clements, M. 'Immunisation and the sudden infant death syndrome', *Archives of Disease in Childhood*, 1995; 73(6): 498–501.

52. Ford, RP, Hassall, IB, Mitchell, EA, Scragg, R, Taylor, BJ, Allen, EM and Stewart, AW. 'Life events, social support and the risk of sudden infant death syndrome', *Journal of Child Psychology and Psychiatry and Allied Disciplines*, 1996; 37(7): 835–40.

53. Parkins, KJ, Poets, CF, O'Brien, LM, Stebbens, VA and Southall, DP. 'Effect of exposure to 15% oxygen on breathing patterns and oxygen saturation in infants; interventional study', *British Medical Journal*, 1998; 316: 887–94.

54. Ward-Platt, MP, Fleming, PJ, Blair, PS, Leach, CEA, Golding, J and Smith, I. 'Danger to babies from air travel must be small', *British Medical Journal*, 1998; 317: 676–8.

55. Gershon, NB and Moon, RY. 'Infant sleep position in licensed child care centers', *Pediatrics*, 1997; 100: 75–8.

56. Mitchell, EA, Thompson, JM, Stewart, AW, Webster, ML, Taylor, BJ, Hassall, IB, Ford, RP, Allen, EM, Scragg, R and Becroft, DM. 'Postnatal depression and SIDS: a prospective study', *Journal of Paediatrics and Child Health*, 1992; 28 (supplement 1): S13–S16.

57. Coghill, SR, Caplan, HL, Alexandra, H *et al.* 'Impact of maternal depression on the cognitive development of young children', *British Medical Journal*, 1986; 292: 1165–7.

58. Holden, JM. 'Postnatal depression: its nature, effects and identification using the Edinburgh Postnatal Depression scale', *Birth*, 1991; 18: 211–21.

59. Stuart, S, Couser, G, Schilder, K, O'Hara, MW and Gorman, L. 'Postpartum anxiety and depression: onset and comorbidity in a community sample', *Journal of Nervous and Mental Disease*, 1998; 186: 420–4.

60. Gilbert, RE, Wigfield, RE, Fleming, PJ, Berry, PJ and Rudd, PT. 'Bottle feeding and the sudden infant death syndrome', *British Medical Journal*, 1995; 310(6972): 88–90.

61. Mitchell, EA. 'Smoking: the next major and modifiable risk factor' in Rognum, TO (ed.) *Sudden Infant Death Syndrome: New Trends in the Nineties*. Oslo: Scandinavian University Press; 1995: 114–18.

62. Alm, B, Milerad, J, Wennergren, G, Skjaerven, R, Oyen, O, Norvenius, G *et al.* 'A case-control study of smoking and sudden infant death syndrome in the Scandinavian countries, 1992 to 1995', *Archives of Disease in Childhood*, 1998; 78: 329–44.

63. Blair, PS, Fleming, PJ, Bensley, D, Smith, I, Bacon, C, Taylor, BJ, Berry, J, Golding, J and Tripp, J. 'Smoking and the sudden infant death syndrome: results from 1993–5 case-control study for confidential enquiry into stillbirths and deaths in infancy', *British Medical Journal*, 1996; 313(7051): 195–8.

64. Cnattingius, S and Nordstrom, M-L. 'Maternal smoking and feto-infant mortality: biological pathways and public health significance', *Acta Paediatrica*, 1996; 85: 1400–2.

65. Gospe, SM, Zhou, SS and Pinkerton, KE. 'Effects of environmental tobacco smoke exposure *in utero* and/or postnatally on brain development', *Pediatric Research*, 1996; 39(3): 494–8.

66. Drews, CD, Murphy, CC, Yeargin-Allsop, M and Decoufle, P. 'The relationship between idiopathic mental retardation and maternal smoking during pregnancy', *Pediatrics*, 1996; 97(4): 547–53.

67. Storm, H, Nylander, G and Saugstad, OD. 'The amount of brainstem gliosis in sudden infant death syndrome (SIDS) victims correlates with maternal cigarette smoking during pregnancy', *Acta Paediatrica*, 1999; 88(1): 13–18.

68. Hill, AB. 'The environment and disease: association or causation?', *Proc. Royal Soc. Med.*, 1965; 58: 295–300.

69. Oyen, N, Haglund, B, Skjaerven, R and Irgens, LM. 'Maternal smoking, birthweight and gestational age in sudden infant death syndrome (SIDS) babies and their surviving siblings', *Paediat. Perinat. Epidemiol.*, 1997; 11 (supplement 1): 1–12.

Chapter 4

The Pathology Study: The Contribution of Ancillary Pathology Tests to the Investigation of Unexpected Infant Death

Jem Berry, Eleanor Allibone, Pat McKeever, Isabella Moore, Chris Wright and Peter Fleming

Results of an analysis of 450 post-mortem reports from the CESDI SUDI study: introduction

Post-mortem examination is a vital part of the investigation of sudden unexpected infant deaths. It is essential for establishing the cause of death in those cases with recognisable illnesses such as pneumonia or meningitis. Equally, a thorough post-mortem examination is necessary to exclude natural or unnatural disease processes that might be responsible for death before SIDS can be given as the 'cause' of death. Occasionally, post-mortem examination demonstrates that an apparently natural death was due to injury. The welcome fall in the SIDS rate which followed the 'Back to Sleep' campaign has resulted in a greater proportion of fully explained deaths in the SUDI population, and so careful post-mortem examination has become more important as cot deaths have become less common.

The definition of SIDS stipulates that no cause of death is found after a 'thorough' post-mortem examination. As knowledge about the possible causes of SUDI has increased, so the number and variety of ancillary laboratory tests recommended in cot death post-mortems has increased [1]. This has met with resistance from some coroners and health care trusts who may be unwilling to meet the financial consequences of these investigations.

There is broad national and international agreement among pathologists with special experience in this field about the tests necessary to exclude common causes of unexpected death in infancy. In addition to routine autopsy, these tests include:

- microscopic examination of tissue samples (histology) to look for evidence of disease such as pneumonia;
- bacteriological examination of blood, cerebrospinal fluid and lung to rule out septicaemia, meningitis and bacterial lung infection, respectively;
- virological examination of the upper and lower respiratory tract and bowel;
- an X-ray of the whole body to exclude unsuspected fractures;
- analysis of the vitreous humour (eye fluid) to detect dehydration;
- examination of a frozen section of liver for fat to screen for the commonest inherited biochemical defect causing SUDI.

These investigations have been widely used in research studies, but there has never been a systematic investigation of their value in routine post-mortem practice. The CESDI study provided a unique opportunity to evaluate their contribution to diagnosis and provide a revised protocol based on the evidence obtained.

Pathologists were asked to carry out their post-mortem examinations to a standard protocol [2] based on that recommended by the Royal College of Pathologists [3], so that at the conclusion of the study it would be possible to analyse reports in a systematic way to evaluate the contribution of ancillary tests to the final post-mortem diagnosis. This chapter describes the results of that analysis and concludes with a suggested 'evidence based' post-mortem protocol.

Pathologists have already contributed to the CESDI SUDI study in several other ways:

- by providing pathology reports and causes of death for epidemiological studies;

- by taking part in confidential enquiry panels;

- by providing samples for antimony analysis in the final year of the study.

Study design

The cooperation of every pathologist in each of the regions taking part in the study was sought by letter, and they were provided with a copy of the CESDI SUDI post-mortem protocol. Training in appropriate autopsy method and interpretation was offered, and financial assistance to meet the cost of performing ancillary tests was provided.

CESDI regional coordinators were asked to supply complete post-mortem reports with the hospital of origin and pathologist's name removed. CESDI regional pathology coordinators were asked to collect spare sets of microscope slides, and these and the reports have been collated into a pathology archive of the CESDI SUDI study.

The post-mortem reports were each analysed by one of the regional pathology coordinators, without knowledge of the final conclusion reached by the local pathologist, using a detailed protocol to ensure consistency.

A pilot study of 100 cases was evaluated initially, and the protocol was then revised in the light of those results. The post-mortem reports for the entire data set were then evaluated, using the revised protocol.

Protocol for assessment of post-mortem investigations and reports

Each report was abstracted sequentially. First, basic demographic data were extracted from the report. Then the clinical history was assessed for adequacy to direct subsequent post-mortem examination and ancillary investigations. The investigations considered necessary based on the history as given in the report were recorded in a structured database. The external and internal examinations were recorded in the same way, and a second decision taken about which investigations were indicated by the findings from the gross post-mortem examination. The additional studies actually undertaken and the results of those tests were then recorded and their contribution to diagnosis scored.

Finally, the cause of death as given by the original pathologist was recorded, and the pathologist who carried out the post-mortem was classified according to grade and discipline (trainee, consultant histopathologist, consultant paediatric pathologist, consultant forensic pathologist), and the completeness of the report recorded.

The findings of the regional pathology coordinator were classified according to the Avon clinico-pathological classification [4]. This gives a measure of the extent to which the autopsy findings provide an explanation for a baby's death. After assessment of all available clinical and pathological information, deaths were placed in one of three broad categories:

I. no significant findings;

II. findings that may have contributed to ill-health and possibly to death;

III. findings that provide a full explanation for death.

Results

Ascertainment

A total of 450 post-mortem reports were received. These included some cases which were not subjected to confidential enquiry because of ongoing police investigation. Because of the importance of maintaining the anonymity of the confidential enquiries, no direct link could be used to provide a comparison between the results of this part of the SUDI study and the confidential enquiry or the case-control study. For some deaths, information which became available from the questionnaire, narrative account, local case discussion meeting or health care records at the time of the confidential enquiry meeting shed new light on the events leading up to the death and led to a change in the identified 'cause' of death. Thus, the distribution of 'causes' of death in the initial pathology reports included in this study is not identical to that described elsewhere in this report. Additional information which may have been available at the confidential enquiry meeting was, for the same reasons, not available to the regional pathology coordinator who carried out the independent review of each post-mortem report. Thus, the final 'cause' of death attributed by the regional pathology coordinator may also have been different to that attributed by the confidential review panel. In particular, the assessment of whether a death initially attributed to trauma or accidental causes was in fact accidental or non-accidental requires additional information which was rarely, if ever, available at the time of the initial post-mortem examination (see Chapter 7).

The collection of pathology reports was, however, virtually complete (450 reports obtained from a maximum possible number of 464 deaths which occurred in the study regions during the period of study: i.e. 97% ascertainment).

Post-mortem interval

Twenty-eight per cent of the examinations were carried out on the day of death, 67% within one day, 81% within two days, 93% within three days, and 98% within four days.

Cause of death

Overall, the cause of death was given as SIDS in 315 (70%) of cases, and non-SIDS in 135 (30%) of cases by the original pathologist. Using the Avon classification, the reviewer assigned 253 (56.2%) to group I (no pathological finding which contributed to death), 117 (26%) to group II (pathological findings which possibly or probably contributed to death) and 80 (17.8%) to group III (death fully explained by the pathological findings).

This equates to 369 out of 450 (82%) SIDS (Avon groups I and II) and 80 out of 450 (17.8%) non-SIDS SUDI (Avon group III). A comparison with the breakdown of 'causes' attributed by the confidential enquiry and the case-control study is given later in this chapter.

Pathologist

Four per cent of examinations were carried out by trainees, 49% by consultant histopathologists, 32% by consultant paediatric pathologists, and 14% by forensic pathologists. The reports of trainees were of a high standard and appeared to be closely supervised and only undertaken at specialist institutions.

Different subspecialties within pathology made different use of ancillary tests, the most being undertaken by paediatric pathologists, and the fewest by forensic pathologists (Table 4.1). However, the latter used toxicology in 8% of cases compared with about 2% for the other specialties. The cause of death was given as unascertained in 16% of cases examined by forensic pathologists, and as due to accident or trauma in a further 14%, reflecting their different case mix compared with non-forensic pathologists. Paediatric pathologists gave the cause of death as SIDS in 76% of cases, general pathologists in 70% and forensic pathologists in 59% of cases.

Table 4.1 Who includes what in their reports? Tests and conclusions reported by different pathology specialties*

	General pathologists (% reported)	Paediatric pathologists (% reported)	Forensic pathologists (% reported)
Some history	95	92	89
X-ray report	53	69	47
Adequate histology	53	69	47
Frozen section report	33	70	8
Vitreous electrolytes	33	70	8
Blood culture report	61	86	19
CSF bacteriology	61	77	23
Lung bacteriology	60	60	22
Lung virology	53	85	9
Toxicology	2	1.4	8
Non-SIDS diagnosis*	30	24	41
Final report	97	94	95

* The percentages of cases not ascribed to SIDS by each specialty is also shown. (CSF = cerebrospinal fluid)

Trends during the three years of the study

During the three years of the study, there was evidence of increased use of paediatric pathologists (24% of examinations in year one, 46% of examinations in year three). The use of ancillary tests also increased. For example, no blood culture was undertaken in 38% of cases in the first year, but only 24% of cases in the third year. Fifty-one per cent of post-mortem examinations in the first year had no evidence of an X-ray, and this figure had decreased to 40% by the third year.

Investigations

Histology

Histology proved the most valuable single ancillary investigation giving positive findings thought relevant to the cause of death in 63 of 404 cases (15.5%) in which the results of histology were recorded.

Histological findings at least probably relevant to death were present in 89 of 404 cases (22%).

In those cases in which there was a significant histological finding responsible for death, the affected organ was predicted correctly by the reviewer from the history alone in 83% of cases. The history indicated the need for histology in a further 11%, but the wrong organ system was predicted from the history. The organ system affected was incorrectly predicted in three cases of myocarditis, two cases of meningitis and one case each of encephalitis and bronchopneumonia.

Histology was not thought to be indicated from the history in only 6% of those cases in which there was a positive finding thought to be responsible for death. These unanticipated histological findings were three cases of lower respiratory tract infection and a case of transverse myelitis.

Abnormal histology can therefore be predicted from the history by an experienced paediatric pathologist in a majority of cases, but it is necessary to carry out histology as a routine if important observations are not to be missed.

Frozen section of liver

Pathologists were asked to carry out a frozen section of liver stained for neutral fat. This examination was recorded as having been carried out in 196 cases. Many other post-mortem reports mentioned the presence or absence of fatty change in the liver without stating that a frozen section had been carried out.

In five of these 196 cases, there was very extensive fatty change. In two cases a diagnosis of medium chain acyl Co-A dehydrogenase (MCAD) deficiency was confirmed biochemically. A third case had galactosaemia, and in a fourth case MCAD deficiency was excluded. The fifth case was a baby who had been maintained on a ventilator following a collapse thought possibly to be due to hyperthermia.

In 87 of the 196 cases, the frozen section was described as showing mild to moderate fatty change. The remainder were either normal or there was no final report. The finding of two cases of MCAD deficiency in 189 frozen sections gives a maximum detection rate of 1.06 per 100 infant deaths. It is likely that the true rate in this study was lower because the result of some frozen sections carried out may not have appeared in the final post-mortem report. On the other hand, it is likely that other cases were missed because frozen sections were not carried out, and indeed a further case of MCAD deficiency was detected by analysis of urine for dicarboxylic acids apparently without frozen section.

Although not requested in the CESDI SUDI post-mortem protocol, a few units carried out some kind of routine biochemical screening in addition to frozen section. No further abnormality was found in 57 cases other than a single case in which salicylate metabolites were detected in a metabolic screen of urine.

There were three cases in which moderate fatty change in the liver was probably over-interpreted, leading to inappropriate suspicion of an inborn error of metabolism.

Bacteriology

Blood cultures: Blood cultures were recorded as having been undertaken in 287 cases. A major pathogen with corresponding histological changes was found in seven cases, or 2.4% of those in which the result of a blood culture was recorded. A further eight cases grew a single pathogenic organism, but without corresponding histology. These organisms were *Staphylococcus aureus* in three cases, group B beta-haemolytic *Streptococcus* in three cases, and two cases with an alpha-haemolytic *Streptococcus*. These two groups in which single organisms were isolated with or without corresponding histology account for nearly 5% of the cases in which the results of blood culture were stated.

Mixed cultures were obtained from 130 cases, and sterile cultures from 144. There was no clear relationship between mixed growth in blood cultures and increasing post-mortem interval.

Cerebrospinal fluid: The result of 279 cultures of cerebrospinal fluid (CSF) were recorded in the post-mortem reports. There were seven positive cultures of CSF associated with corresponding histological changes in the brain. The organisms were *Neisseria meningitidis* (three cases), *Haemophilus influenzae* type B, *Escherichia coli*, group A beta-haemolytic *Streptococcus*, and *Staphylococcus epidermidis* (one case each).

In a further 10 cases, a single potential pathogen was grown from CSF without corresponding histological changes in the brain. These organisms included *N. meningitidis*, *Streptococcus pneumoniae* (two cases), haemolytic *Streptococcus* (three cases) and *Haemophilus* (two cases). In most of these cases, the organism was also isolated from other sites, and in several was associated with a significant respiratory tract infection. In 51 other cases there was a growth of mixed organisms or a single organism considered to be a contaminant. In 211 cases, the CSF was sterile.

The rate of isolation of a single pathogen with associated central nervous system histological abnormalities was 2.5%. The rate of isolation of a single pathogen with or without histological changes in the brain was 6%.

Lung bacteriology: Interpretation of bacteriology of the respiratory tract is complicated by the presence of commensal organisms, some of which may be pathogens in certain circumstances. Results were available from 233 lung cultures, although more had clearly been taken and the results not recorded.

In eight cases, there was a clear association between a major pathogen and significant histological changes in the lungs. These pathogens were *Haemophilus influenzae*, *Streptococcus pneumoniae* (two cases), *Staphylococcus aureus* (two cases) and *Bordetella pertussis* (one case). In a further 27 cases, a potential pathogen was isolated from the lung, but was associated with minor or no histological changes. Sometimes the same organism was isolated from multiple sites, or occasionally was part of a generalised septicaemia. In 117 further cases, organisms were interpreted as normal flora or contaminants. In 81 cases, lung cultures were recorded as negative.

A major pathogen was associated with significant histological changes in the lungs in 3.4%. Fifteen per cent of cases had a single potential major pathogen isolated from lung tissue with or without corresponding histopathological findings.

Virology

Nasopharyngeal aspirate: Viruses were detected in five of 112 or 4.5% of nasopharyngeal aspirates in which the results were recorded. In four of the five cases, the virus was associated with significant histological changes (Table 4.2).

Lung virology: Viruses were detected in 11 of 264 (4.2%) of samples of lung tissue. In nine of these, there was significant pathology that was attributable to the virus. In two cases, a polio virus, presumed to be a vaccine strain, was isolated (Table 4.3).

Gastro-intestinal virology: Viruses were isolated from 43 of 237 (18%) of cases in which reports were available. In three of these, the viruses were associated with significant pathology, none associated directly with the gastro-intestinal tract (Table 4.4). In 40 further cases, the significance of the virus isolates was doubtful (Table 4.5). Twenty-two samples yielded polio viruses, presumed to be vaccine strains. None of the cases in which viruses were isolated from the gastro-intestinal tract were associated with a history suggesting gastro-enteritis. In one case, the vitreous sodium was 153 mmol/l, the bowel was empty and a polio virus was isolated. In others, the virus may have been the cause of a minor systemic upset.

Table 4.2 Viruses isolated from 112 nasopharyngeal aspirates in which the results were given

Virus	Associated pathology
RSV	Tracheobronchitis
RSV	Lymphocytic tracheitis
Coxsackie B2	Myocarditis
Rhinovirus	Tracheobronchitis
Parainfluenza	None

Table 4.3 Viruses isolated from 264 lung specimens in which the results were known

Virus	Associated pathology
RSV	Bronchiolitis
RSV	Bronchiolitis
Paraflu 3	Mild lymphocytic tracheitis
Paraflu 1	Necrotising tracheitis
Herpes 1	Neonatal herpes simplex infection
CMV	Encephalitis and myocarditis
CMV	Lymphocytic infiltrate in lung and trachea
Echovirus 22	Lymphocytic tracheobronchiolitis
Coxsackie B5	Transverse myelitis
Polio 1*	–
Polio 2*	–

* Presumed vaccine strains

Table 4.4 Viruses isolated from the gastro-intestinal tract with significant associated pathology

Virus	Associated pathology
Coxsackie B2	Myocarditis
Coxsackie B1	Transverse myelitis
HSV 1	Neonatal HSV infection

237 cases with reports

Vitreous electrolytes

The results of analysis of vitreous humour for electrolytes were available in 179 cases. Mean values for sodium and urea concentrations remained remarkably constant until the fourth day after death, when the sodium concentration apparently fell (Table 4.6). The potassium level rose rapidly after death.

Table 4.5 Positive gastro-intestinal virology not associated with significant clinical illness or pathology

Polio*	22
Rotavirus	5
Adenovirus	4
Echovirus	4
Coxsackie virus	3
Enterovirus (not specified)	2

40 of 237 cases with reports

* Presumed vaccine strains

Table 4.6 Mean vitreous electrolyte values (mmol/litre) and post-mortem interval

Post-mortem interval	Sodium	Urea	Potassium
0 days	139	4.5	12.3
1 day	138	5.0	17.8
2 days	135	5.8	21.8
3 days	129	5.9	31.5
4 days	125	5.3	29.6

The highest values (sodium 166, urea 7.5 mmol/l) were recorded in a four-week-old baby with *E. coli* septicaemia and peritonitis. No case of death definitely attributable to dehydration was ascertained from vitreous electrolytes, but cases with moderately raised levels are listed in Table 4.7. Thirty cases in which results were available had vitreous sodium levels of 130 mmol/l or less, 22 of these with values less than 120 mmol/l. These cases had no particular clinical features and came from all five health care regions in the study. It is possible that these low results are a result of a technical problem in sampling viscous fluids through the fine tubing of modern auto-analysers.

Table 4.7 Abnormally high vitreous electrolyte levels (mmol/litre)

Sodium	Urea	Clinical features
166	7.5	*Escherichia coli* septicaemia and peritonitis
158	7.7	5-month-old found 'wet with sweat'
153	4.2	Failure to thrive; empty bowel
151	7.3	Failure to thrive; delay calling ambulance
151	6.8	6-day-old dead in bed in mother's arms
150	10.9	Aborted SIDS with brain damage

Vitreous glucose estimation was not included in the CESDI protocol, but results were available in 86 cases. The vitreous glucose level was < 0.5 mmol/l in 73% of cases.

Radiology

Two hundred and fifty-three cases were recorded as having been X-rayed prior to post-mortem examination. Two hundred and forty-six of these X-rays were commented on in the post-mortem reports. There were five cases in which healing fractures were detected. Three had healing posterior rib fractures, and one a healing fracture of the femur. One other case had healing rib fractures and multiple Wormian bones attributed to osteogenesis inperfecta. Four of these five cases were still attributed to SIDS despite the fractures, and one death was attributed to blunt head injury. In the case of the blunt head injury, the rib fractures were diagnosed after exhumation prompted by injury of a sibling. In four of the five cases in which bony injury was demonstrated by radiology, the investigation was indicated by the history. In the fifth, a healing rib fracture found at the post-mortem examination indicated the need for skeletal survey.

Positive findings of doubtful significance were found in a further 25 cases, including physiological periosteal reaction in six, suspicion of intramural gas in the bowel in two (not confirmed by direct examination of the bowel), pneumoperitoneum, pneumothorax and gas in the portal vein (all thought to be due to resuscitation or post-mortem change). In one case, a radio-opaque button was observed in the stomach of a baby with recurrent apnoeic spells whose sibling subsequently died unexpectedly and whose mother was subsequently convicted of causing the death.

Rectal temperature

The measurement of rectal temperature at the time the infant was found, or on arrival at hospital, was not part of the post-mortem protocol. However, it was recorded in 27 reports. The rectal temperature was more than 38° C in 10 of these cases, and more than 39° C in six cases. The highest recorded rectal temperature was 41° C. Of the six babies with a rectal temperature greater than 39° C, three were found completely under their bedding, one drenched in sweat. A further baby was almost certainly overwrapped, and its bedding was also described as wet.

How do ancillary tests influence the cause of death?

Ancillary tests when the cause of death was other than SIDS

In 132 cases, the cause of death was given as something other than SIDS or an equivalent by the original pathologist. The investigations indicating the major cause of death or probable contributory causes are listed in Table 4.8.

Table 4.8 Ancillary tests indicating major or probable contributory cause of death

	Major cause of death	Probable contributory cause	Total
Histology	59	10	69
Bacteriology	16	6	22
Virology	6	1	7
Frozen section of liver	2	0	2 *
X-ray	0	2 [†]	2 [†]
Vitreous electrolytes	0	0	0

132 cases not ascribed to SIDS

* Medium chain acyl Co-A dehydrogenase deficiency confirmed, a third case in this group was diagnosed by analysis of urine

[†] Old posterior rib fractures confirmed by histology

Histology was the single most useful investigation, and the respiratory tract the organ system most often found to be abnormal (Table 4.9). It was clear that significant pathology in the lungs such as bronchiolitis could not be predicted reliably from macroscopic examination. There was almost certainly over-interpretation of normal microscopic features of infant lung, such as peribronchial lymphoid aggregates, and some deaths were probably incorrectly attributed to aspiration of gastric contents. Examination of the central nervous system showed conditions such as meningitis, encephalitis, unsuspected transverse myelitis, micropolygyria, ischaemic changes and trauma. Histology of the heart showed myocarditis, cardiomyopathy, rhabdomyomas and post-resuscitation infarction. In the gastro-intestinal system, there was enteritis, colitis and ischaemic damage due to intussusception and 'near-miss events'. The commonest change in the endocrine system was adrenal haemorrhage characteristic of Waterhouse–Friderichsen syndrome. In the genito-urinary system, the most frequent abnormality was cytomegalovirus in renal tubules, which in some cases was part of a significant infection.

These results provide little or no support for routine retention of the whole heart or brain in the absence of focal lesions or a suggestive history. The only finding which would have been missed was a single case of unsuspected transverse myelitis.

Table 4.9 Positive histology (major or probable contributory cause of death) by organ system

Organ system	Number of cases with positive histology
Respiratory tract	46
Central nervous system	27
Heart	10
Gastro-intestinal	13
Endocrine	5
Genito-urinary	5
Skeletal	2
Skin *	1

132 SUDIs not ascribed to SIDS

* Hypohydrotic ectodermal dysplasia

Bacteriology established the major cause of death in 16 cases, and a probable contributory cause in six. Virology gave a major or probable contributory cause of death in seven cases. It was notable that the responsible organism was not always isolated from the site of pathology, but from a related or distant site. Bacteriology of gastro-intestinal contents was not part of the CESDI protocol, but revealed *Campylobacter* in one case with gastro-enteritis, and *Clostridium difficile* with histological evidence of pseudo-membranous colitis in another.

Positive pathology tests in fully explained deaths

On review, 80 of the 450 cases were considered to fall into group III of the Avon classification (death fully explained by findings, Table 4.10). This group excluded those cases in which the cause of death given by the original pathologist was considered to be less than a full explanation for death, and cases in which death was ascribed to hypoxic-ischaemic brain damage secondary to an unexplained 'near-miss' event. Other cases were reassigned on the basis of the structured, standardised review by the regional CESDI pathology coordinators.

Histology was the single most useful investigation and was positive in 67% (Table 4.11). The contribution of the other tests to determining the cause of death is listed.

When histology was positive, the respiratory tract was the most frequent site, closely followed by the central nervous system. The number of significant positive histological findings is given in Table 4.12.

Table 4.10 Cause of death in Avon group III cases

Organ system	Cause of death	Number of cases
Respiratory	Bronchiolitis	5
	Pneumonia	14
Central nervous system	Meningitis	4
	Encephalitis	2
	Trauma	10
	Vascular malformation	1
Cardiovascular	Myocarditis	4
	Cardiomyopathy	1
	Congenital	10
Gastro-intestinal	Intussusception	2
	Volvulus	1
	Gastro-enteritis/colitis	3
Septicaemia (without meningitis)	Menningococcus	4
	Escherichia coli	2
	Waterhouse–Friderichsen (no organism isolated)	2
Accident/trauma (excluding head injury)	Hanging/wedging	5
	Choking	2
	Drowning	2
	Other	1
Metabolic	MCAD	3
Other	Neonatal herpes simplex	1
	Ectodermal dysplasia	1
		n = 80

* The immediate cause of death is given, some babies in the respiratory group having underlying congenital disorders

MCAD, medium chain acyl Co-A dehydrogenase deficiency

Table 4.11 Ancillary tests indicating the major or probable contributory cause of death

	Major cause of death	Probable contributor to death	Total	%
Histology	49	5	54	67
Bacteriology	17	2	19	11
Virology	5	0	5	6.25
Frozen section	3	0	3	3.75
X-ray	2	1	3	3.75
Vitreous electrolytes	0	0	0	0

80 cases in which death was fully explained (Avon classification group III)

Table 4.12 Positive histology indicating the major or probable contributory cause of death by organ system

Organ system	Number of cases with positive histology
Respiratory tract	20
Central nervous system	16
Cardiovascular system	8
Gastro-intestinal	6
Endocrine (adrenal)	5
Genito-urinary	1
Skeletal	3

80 cases in which death was fully explained (Avon classification group III)

A comparison of the 'causes' of death given for SUDI by the confidential enquiry, local pathologists and regional paediatric pathologists

The conclusions reached by the professionals involved in each part of the study (case-control, confidential enquiry, pathology) about the 'causes' of deaths of the infants in the study show some discrepancies, but as noted above and in Chapters 3 and 5, these arose because of different information being available at different times during the process of the investigations. In addition, because of potential legal and confidentiality issues, the confidential enquiry and case-control parts of the study excluded many infants whose deaths were initially suspected as being due to or subsequently attributed to non-accidental injury (including suffocation). Despite these limitations, the final conclusions of the local case discussion meeting, the confidential enquiry panel, and the regional pathology coordinator's review were in general agreement as to the broad grouping of 'causes' of the deaths – at least as far as their classification into SIDS and non-SIDS is concerned. As noted above, the major limitation of the assessment by the regional pathology coordinators was the lack of information concerning the circumstances of the death and family background, which were important factors for both the local case discussion meetings and the confidential enquiry in assessing whether deaths were accidental or non-accidental. This particularly applied to those deaths attributed by the confidential enquiry panels to probable or possible smothering by a parent. A summary of the overall classification of the 'causes' of the deaths from the different parts of the CESDI SUDI study is given in Table 4.13. Because of the anonymisation of records prior to the confidential enquiry process, it is not possible to make a direct comparison of the conclusions of the confidential enquiry with those of the regional pathology reviewers for individual cases. The high level of ascertainment for both the pathology and the case-control studies (97% and 98%, respectively) allows overall comparisons to be made between these two studies.

From this table, it can be seen that the initial assessments of the local pathologists (which would usually be incorporated into the registered causes of death) were substantially different from all other assessments. As noted above, the local pathologists sometimes attributed deaths to 'causes' which were not considered as sufficient causes of death by an expert paediatric pathologist. However, this possible 'misclassification' of deaths at the initial post-mortem examination involved both an over-interpretation of relatively minor pathological changes and a failure to identify the significance of real pathology (e.g. fractures). The real level of discrepancy between the attributed causes of death between the local pathologists and the regional reviewers was thus greater than the overall figures would suggest. These findings are remarkably similar to those of the Knowelden study of post–neonatal deaths in the 1970s [5].

Table 4.13 A comparison of the 'causes' of death given for sudden unexpected deaths in infancy by different groups in the CESDI SUDI study

'Cause' of death attributed by:	Number of SUDI included**	% of total	Deaths attrib- uted to SIDS††	% of total	Deaths attributed to Non-SIDS SUDI‡‡	% of total
	n	%	n	%	n	%
Local pathologist*	450	97	315	70	135	30
Regional pathology coordinator§	450	97	369	82	80	18
Confidential enquiry†	417	90†	346	83	71	17
Confidential enquiry or local case discussion‡	456	98	363	80	93	20

* Cause of death given on the post-mortem report (see above). Usually the same as the registered cause of death, but information on the registered cause of death was not separately collected in this study

† The conclusion reached for those cases subjected to a confidential enquiry. Those cases initially suspected of being due to non-accidental injury (NAI) were excluded from the confidential enquiry

‡ In the case-control study, some infants were included for whom no confidential enquiry meeting took place (as noted above). For these cases, the assessment of 'cause' of death was taken as that attributed by the local case discussion meeting. Because of the exclusion of suspected non-accidental injury from the confidential enquiry procedure, this classification includes slightly more 'explained' deaths (mostly NAI) than the confidential enquiry result (see Chapter 3)

§ The assessment reached by the regional pathology coordinators after structured review of the post-mortem results (see above)

** The total number of deaths which occurred in the study regions during the period of the study (as ascertained by the Office for National Statistics) was 464 (see Chapter 3). The percentage ascertainment is based on this figure

††Defined as groups I and II in the Avon clinico-pathological classification [4], i.e. deaths for which no full explanation was found (see above and Chapters 1 and 3)

‡‡Defined as group III in the Avon clinico-pathological classification [4], i.e. deaths for which a full explanation was found (see above and Chapters 1 and 3)

The similarities between the results of the paediatric pathologists' review and the confidential enquiry panels may reflect to some extent the consistent involvement of the regional paediatric pathology coordinators in the confidential enquiry panels.

Conclusion

Perhaps the single most useful component of the investigation of sudden unexpected death in infancy is a very detailed clinical history, which should include if possible a detailed description of the precise circumstances of the death. This will not only point to cases with a complete explanation for death prior to autopsy, but in some cases indicates the organ system that requires particularly careful investigation.

It is not always possible even for experienced pathologists to recognise pulmonary infection or fatty change in the liver from macroscopic appearances, or predict which cases will have positive cultures of blood or cerebrospinal fluid. This confirms the necessity of following a protocol in carrying out post-mortem examinations of infants who have died suddenly and unexpectedly.

Histology was the single most useful ancillary investigation, and so is recommended in every case. Samples should be taken from the upper and lower respiratory tract, including all five lobes of the lungs. Positive and diagnostic pathology is also frequent in the heart and brain.

A frozen section of liver for fat is currently the most easily available screening test for MCAD, and should be undertaken in every case. Residual tissue should be saved as a source of DNA analysis in case the frozen section is positive.

Bacteriology either led to or confirmed the diagnosis in a significant proportion of cases. Single organisms were grown from the blood in 5% of cases. The addition of a carefully taken routine culture of spleen to the protocol would help to confirm the significance of an organism in blood in the absence of associated histological changes. Tracheal bacteriology generally yielded mixed organisms and was unhelpful in the absence of macroscopic pathology. It is recommended that culture of blood, cerebrospinal fluid, lung and a spleen swab should be routine investigations, and additional bacteriological samples be taken where indicated by macroscopic findings. A long post-mortem interval is not a reason for not attempting bacteriology.

Virology demonstrated an organism responsible for or contributing to death in 3.7% of cases. Samples from the respiratory tract (nasopharyngeal aspirate or lung) were often helpful, while many organisms isolated from the gastro-intestinal tract were either polio viruses of presumed vaccine strain, or viruses that were not relevant to the child's death. Occasionally, the virus responsible for a distant lesion such as myocarditis was isolated only from bowel contents. Routine virological sampling of the upper and lower respiratory tract is necessary in view of the difficulty of recognising significant pathology macroscopically. Routine sampling of bowel contents is not supported by this study because of the very high rate of isolation of incidental viruses. Sampling should be restricted to those cases with symptoms related to the gastro-intestinal tract, autopsy findings suggestive of gastro-enteritis, and cases in which the history or post-mortem indicate a significant systemic illness.

Vitreous electrolytes did not demonstrate a single case of unsuspected dehydration or salt poisoning. However, results confirmed the stability of sodium and urea values for several days after death, and that mild dehydration is a common association of systemic illness and a possible contributor to death. The significance of occasional low sodium levels is unknown, but may well be an artefact. Very low levels of glucose in the vitreous humour are extremely common, and there is no evidence that they indicate ante-mortem hypoglycaemia. (High values may be significant and indicate hyperglycaemia prior to death, but are rare in infancy.)

Routine radiology demonstrated fractures in less than 2% of cases in which this was undertaken. In all of these cases, radiological examination was indicated by the history, or a fracture was found at post-mortem examination, prompting skeletal survey. A concern was that in all but one case where there was also blunt injury to the head, death was attributed to natural causes. It is important that X-rays are reviewed by an experienced radiologist, and that any fractures are drawn to the attention of somebody experienced in child abuse.

There have been several developments in the field of unexpected infant death since the original CESDI SUDI post-mortem protocol was devised.

- The CESDI investigation itself has demonstrated the frequency of drug abuse among parents whose children die suddenly and unexpectedly. There is no European study demonstrating a significant incidence of poisoning by recreational or therapeutic drugs in babies who die suddenly and unexpectedly. Nevertheless, consideration should be given to toxicological analyses in individual cases, and appropriate samples should ideally be retained as a routine in case questions are raised later.

- Recent work has suggested that the finding of abundant intra-alveolar haemosiderin in the lungs of babies who die suddenly and unexpectedly can be associated with episodes of previous imposed upper airway obstruction. A section of lung stained by Perls' Prussian blue method may be a useful screening test which may alert the pathologist in some cases, but does not exclude suffocation in others.

- Measurement of the rectal temperature as soon as death is certified may help clarify the physiological mechanism of death when there is no finding at post-mortem examination. However, there are no data available about the normal behaviour of body temperature after death in infants.

Sudden infant death syndrome is a diagnosis of exclusion. In this context, negative results are positive findings. SIDS is now less common than formerly, and so the proportion of explained natural and unnatural deaths among the cot death population has increased. In this study, 17% of deaths were fully explained by postmortem, and this is probably a minimum figure. The findings in cases in which a full range of ancillary tests was undertaken demonstrate the likelihood that causes of death were missed in those in which tests were not carried out. The percentage of positive results for each test in which the result was recorded is given in Table 4.14. These figures represent the maximum chance of missing a significant result if these tests are not carried out.

Table 4.14 Ancillary tests: percentage of significant positive results in those cases in which the result was recorded

Ancillary test	Positive results %
Histology	15.5–22
Blood culture (single organism plus/minus abnormal histology)	2.4–5
CSF (single organism plus/minus abnormal histology)	2.5–6
NPA/lung virology	4.5
X-ray (healing fractures)	2
Frozen section of liver (MCAD deficiency)	1

CSF, cerebrospinal fluid; MCAD, medium chain acyl Co-A dehydrogenase

The importance of full investigation and documentation, including negative findings, may only become apparent when a subsequent child dies, either of natural or unnatural causes. A suggested protocol based on the analysis of the ancillary investigations undertaken in these 450 cases, and their influence on the final diagnosis, is given below (Table 4.15).

Table 4.15 An 'evidence-based' protocol for post-mortem examination of sudden unexpected infant deaths

Full history	Birth history
	Medical history
	Social history
	Health and events preceding death
	Exact circumstances of death
Full autopsy	All body cavities
Full histology	Five lobes of lung, upper and lower respiratory tract
	All major organ systems
	Any lesion
Bacteriology	Blood
	Cerebrospinal fluid
	Lung
	Spleen swab
	Any lesion
Virology	Nasopharyngeal aspirate
	Lung
	Bowel contents (if indicated by history or post-mortem findings)
Vitreous electrolytes	(Sodium and urea)
	Omit if eyes needed for histology (e.g. retinal haemorrhage)
Frozen section of liver for fat	All cases
	Save frozen liver
X-ray	Either all cases, or any cases in which history or
	post-mortem suggests trauma
Consider	Rectal temperature
	Lung section stained by Perls' method
	Toxicology
	Skin, muscle, costochondral junction
	Fibroblast culture

References

1. Krous, HF. 'The international standardised autopsy protocol for sudden unexpected infant death' in Rognum, TO (ed.) *Sudden Infant Death Syndrome: New Trends in the Nineties*. Oslo: Scandinavian University Press, 1995: 81–95.

2. Department of Health. 'Additional guidelines for postmortem investigation associated with studies of sudden infant deaths' in *The Confidential Enquiry into Stillbirths and Deaths in Infancy: First Report*. London: DoH, 1993: appendix F, annex C.

3. Royal College of Pathologists. *Guidelines for Postmortem Examinations after Sudden Unexpected Deaths in Infancy*. London: RCP, 1993.

4. Gilbert, R, Rudd, P, Berry, PJ, Fleming, PJ, Hall, E *et al*. 'Combined effect of infection and heavy wrapping on the risk of sudden infant death', *Archives of Diseases in Childhood*, 1992; 67: 171–7.

5. Knowelden, J, Keeling, J and Nicholl, JP. *A Multicentre Study of Post-neonatal Mortality*. University of Sheffield: Medical Care Research Unit, 1984.

Chapter 5

RESULTS OF CONFIDENTIAL ENQUIRIES

Chris Bacon and John Tripp

SUB-OPTIMAL CARE

Introduction

Confidential enquiries were undertaken in 417 cases, of which 346 were SIDS and 71 were explained deaths, as categorised by the Avon system of classification (Chapter 2). An outline of the procedure for the confidential enquiries is given in Chapter 2; a fuller description and initial results appeared in the Third Annual Report for CESDI [1].

A detailed comparison of the 'causes' of deaths attributed by the three parts of the SUDI study (the case-control study, the pathology study and the confidential enquiry) together with a comparison with the 'causes' initially given by the pathologist who carried out the post-mortem examination is given in Chapter 4.

This chapter concentrates on the instances of sub-optimal care by professionals or by carers that panels identified throughout the three years of the study as possibly or probably contributing to the death of the baby. In the analysis, figures for SIDS and for explained deaths are tabulated separately.

Limitations of the enquiry

In interpreting these findings, it must be borne in mind that the panels did not have the benefit of control cases or of defined standards for good care, and that their assessments were inevitably subjective. The panel validation study [2] showed that there were sometimes inconsistencies between different panels in assessing the same cases. Some panels appeared to be harsher in their judgements than others, particularly with regard to the behaviour of carers. Assessments of professional care were more consistent, being guided by the views of the corresponding panel member on the best standards of current practice. In this context, it would have been an advantage if panel membership had included a social worker. Despite these limitations, we believe that the aggregated conclusions of expert panels on such a large number of cases provide valid guidance on where and how care might be improved.

Number of cases with sub-optimal care

Sub-optimal care was identified in 210 of the 346 SIDS cases and in 37 of the 71 deaths that were explained (Table 5.1). In other words, the panels thought that 61% of SIDS and 52% of explained deaths might possibly have been avoided if professionals or carers had behaved differently. Or, looking at the figures from another way, they thought that nearly half the explained deaths and over a third of the cases of SIDS could not reasonably have been avoided. In many cases, more than one instance of sub-optimal care was identified, often involving professionals and carers together. Factors involving carers were cited in a higher proportion of SIDS, while factors involving professionals were cited in a higher proportion of explained deaths.

Sub-optimal care by professionals

Table 5.2 shows the number of cases in which various professional groups delivered care that panels considered to be sub-optimal. Since most SIDS deaths occur at home it is to be expected that the professionals most often involved will be the primary care team, namely health visitors and general practitioners. Babies dying from disease are more likely to have come to the attention of the general practitioner or of a paediatrician, so that medical care came under scrutiny more often in the explained group. Involvement of obstetricians as well as paediatricians reflects the increased mortality among babies with previous health problems, while involvement of social workers in cases of SIDS reflects its associations with social deprivation and with the possibility of abuse.

Table 5.1 Cases with sub-optimal care

Group involved	SIDS		Explained deaths	
	n	%	n	%
Professionals only	23	6.6	12	16.9
Carers only	123	35.5	17	23.9
Professionals and carers	64	18.5	8	11.3
Total with sub-optimal care	210	60.7	37	52.1
Total with no sub-optimal care	136	39.3	34	47.9
Overall total	346	100	71	100

Table 5.2 Professionals involved in sub-optimal care

Professional group	SIDS		Explained deaths	
	n = 346	%	n = 71	%
Health visitors	40	11.6	6	8.5
General practitioners	29	8.4	14	19.7
Paediatricians	34	9.8	10	14.1
Obstetricians	5	1.4	2	2.8
Hospital midwives	3	0.9	1	1.4
Community midwives	5	1.4	2	2.8
Children's nurses	0	0	2	2.8
Casualty doctors	3	0.9	1	1.4
Casualty nurse	1	0.3	0	0
CONI nurse	1	0.3	0	0
Physiotherapist	1	0.3	0	0
Ambulance staff	0	0	1	1.4
Social workers	21	6.1	0	0

CONI, care of the next infant

Sub-optimal care by health visitors

Since health visitors are required to see all families with new babies, they are the group most exposed to criticism when death occurs unexpectedly at home. Sub-optimal care by health visitors was noted in 40 (12%) cases of SIDS, 61 instances being identified in all. Health visitors were also criticised with regard to some of the explained deaths. Details of the instances in which panels thought that sub-optimal care by the health visitor might have contributed to the death of the baby are given in Table 5.3.

Table 5.3 Sub-optimal care by health visitors

Area of concern	*Instances*			
	SIDS		*Explained deaths*	
	n = 346	*%*	*n = 71*	*%*
Inadequate contact or support	21	6.1	2	2.8
Inadequate advice	16	4.6	0	0
Failure to make medical referral	10	2.9	4	5.6
Failure to monitor baby's weight	4	1.2	0	0
Failure to recognise or act on maternal depression	4	1.2	1	1.4
Failure to recognise risk of abuse	3	0.9	0	0
Poor record keeping	1	0.3	0	0
Poor communication with general practitioner	1	0.3	0	0
Poor communication with social worker	1	0.3	0	0
Total	61	17.6	7	9.9

The most frequent criticism was inadequacy of visits. This usually arose when the health visitor had not given extra support in a case of particular need, for example, if the baby was vulnerable or the mother immature or the home circumstances very poor. Advice might be regarded as inadequate if some aspect of the mother's care was faulty, for example, putting the baby to sleep prone, and there was no record that the health visitor had tried to correct her. Health visitors were criticised on 14 occasions for not referring the case to the general practitioner when they should have been aware that the baby had a problem requiring medical attention; in four of these cases, the problem was urgent and led to the baby's death. Other areas attracting criticism in more than one instance were failure to weigh babies often enough, to arrange help for mothers with depression and to recognise risk of abuse.

Sub-optimal care by general practitioners

Sub-optimal care by general practitioners was identified in 29 (8%) cases of SIDS and 14 (20%) explained deaths, 60 instances being cited in all. Details are given in Table 5.4. The commonest criticism in respect of SIDS, corresponding with that of health visitors, was the failure to recognise that a particular baby was vulnerable and to give adequate medical supervision. For explained deaths, the area that most frequently gave rise to concern was failure to recognise the severity of a baby's illness. General practitioners were also criticised on five occasions for not responding to depression in the mother, and twice for not paying sufficient attention to social problems. In four instances, the records kept by the general practitioner were deemed to be so poor as possibly to have contributed to the baby's death, on the grounds that another doctor seeing the baby was not sufficiently alerted to previous concerns. In many other cases, no assessment of the general practice records was possible because they were not made available to the panel. There were four criticisms for failing to see a baby when the request, in the opinion of the panel, should have received priority, and four for giving mothers advice that was incorrect or inadequate. In five of the explained deaths, the management of the final illness by the general practitioner was thought to have been faulty.

EXAMPLE 1 *(Note: in this example and those that follow, some details have been changed to protect confidentiality, but the essential points remain.)*

A three-month-old girl was abandoned by her mother and left in the care of her father, who was unemployed, took various illegal drugs and led a chaotic life style. The social services department was alerted, who put the baby on the Child Protection Register. The health visitor visited frequently and recorded a fall-off in weight from the 50th to below the 10th centile over the next few months. The baby then developed a respiratory infection and was given antibiotics, but died unexpectedly at home. No significant abnormalities were found at autopsy and the death was registered as SIDS.

The panel thought that the baby's death probably arose from low standards of care. The health visitor was criticised for failing to take action over the poor weight gain that she had documented.

EXAMPLE 2

A six-week-old girl developed a cough and was taken to the general practitioner. He examined the baby and prescribed an antibiotic, and asked the health visitor to visit next day to check her progress. When the health visitor called, the mother pointed out that the baby was breathing faster than usual; she was drowsy and had been unable to take her medicine. The health visitor advised that she should be taken back to the surgery the next day if there was no improvement. Later that evening, the baby abruptly deteriorated and died on the way to hospital. Autopsy revealed widespread staphylococcal pneumonia.

While recognising that staphylococcal infection may progress very rapidly, the panel thought that the health visitor had failed to appreciate the severity of the baby's illness at the time of her visit.

EXAMPLE 3

A boy aged three months had been previously healthy, but then began to vomit, and stopped passing faeces and urine. The vomit became green and specks of blood appeared in the nappy. The general practitioner was called during the night but found no abnormality. The vomiting continued, and the general practitioner was called again the next day, when he prescribed Gaviscon. Forty-eight hours after the onset of the vomiting, the baby became very ill and was taken direct to hospital. Laparotomy revealed intussusception and extensive necrosis. Despite surgery and life support the baby died.

The panel concluded that the death could have been avoided if the general practitioner had recognised the typical features of intussusception at an earlier stage.

Table 5.4   Sub-optimal care by general practitioners

Area of concern	Instances			
	SIDS		Explained deaths	
	n = 346	%	n = 71	%
Failure to recognise vulnerability of baby and/or to provide adequate medical supervision	15	4.3	0	0
Failure to recognise severity of acute illness	4	1.2	10	14.1
Failure to recognise or act on maternal depression	5	1.4	0	0
Inadequate or incorrect advice	4	1.2	0	0
Poor record keeping	4 *	–	0	0
Failure to see baby when requested	2	0.6	2	2.8
Failure to appreciate social problems	1	0.3	2	2.8
Failure to recognise risk of abuse	2	0.6	0	0
Poor communication	1	0.3	1	1.4
Poor relationship with family	1	0.3	0	0
Incorrect clinical management	1	0.3	5	7.0
Total	40	11.6	20	28.2

*   Based on sample only

EXAMPLE 4

A young single mother took her three-month-old baby boy to her doctor in the morning because he felt very hot and had a skin temperature of over 40°C, was off his feeds and had sticky eyes. The doctor examined the baby briefly and prescribed eye drops. Later in the day, the baby began to vomit repeatedly and became very drowsy. The mother called the practice and was told to come at the end of evening surgery. She took the baby straight away nevertheless, but by the time the doctor was free to see him he was limp and unresponsive. The mother was told to take him to hospital in her car; she was delayed and when she arrived the baby was dead. Autopsy showed septicaemia with adrenal haemorrhage.

The panel considered that the general practitioner was at fault for not recognising the severity of the baby's illness when he saw him that morning, and for not calling an ambulance when he saw him again later.

Sub-optimal care by paediatricians

Panels thought that sub-optimal care by paediatricians might have contributed to 34 cases (10%) of SIDS and 10 (14%) explained deaths, citing 40 and 15 instances respectively (Table 5.5). The apparently large number of criticisms of secondary care for deaths that occurred at home reflects the fact that in many cases of SIDS there is a pre-existing medical problem that contributes to the death without being the whole cause. Failures to recognise the severity of illness preceding an explained death usually involved a less experienced doctor who was inadequately supervised. In both SIDS and the explained group, there were criticisms for inadequate investigation, poor clinical management and unsatisfactory arrangements for discharge or follow-up. Paediatricians were criticised on nine occasions for their failure to recognise or act upon a risk of abuse. Although other health professionals may also have been involved, the paediatrician was singled out for criticism because he or she was expected to take the lead on this issue. In three cases, lack of leadership by the paediatrician was specifically mentioned. There were four criticisms of poor communication; these arose when the paediatrician had failed to discuss concerns about a vulnerable baby directly with the general practitioner, relying instead on written reports that were delayed or not sufficiently informative.

Table 5.5 Sub-optimal care by paediatricians

Area of concern	Instances			
	SIDS		Explained deaths	
	n = 346	%	n = 71	%
Poor clinical management	9	2.6	3	4.2
Failure to recognise severity of illness	1	0.3	5	7.0
Inadequate investigation	7	2.0	3	4.2
Poor discharge arrangements	2	0.6	1	1.4
Inadequate follow-up	6	1.7	0	0
Failure to take account of social background	0	0	2	2.8
Failure to recognise or act upon risk of abuse	9	2.6	0	0
Lack of leadership	3	0.9	0	0
Poor communication with general practitioner	3	0.9	1	1.4
Total	40	11.6	15	21.1

EXAMPLE 5

A baby girl was admitted to hospital at the age of six months because she seemed to be generally unwell. She was found to be hypoglycaemic and responded to treatment with intravenous glucose. She was sent home after 48 hours without further investigations. The parents were not advised on her feeding regime but were asked to test her blood glucose at intervals, for which equipment was provided. A few days later, they found a blood glucose of 2 mmol/l in the evening and brought her back to hospital. She was normoglycaemic after a feed and was sent back home again. A week later, she was found dead in her cot at night, having apparently been normal and healthy through the day. No significant abnormalities were found at autopsy, but tests for metabolic abnormality were incomplete. The death was registered as SIDS.

The panel thought that this baby might not have died if her recurrent hypoglycaemia had been adequately investigated and treated. The consultant paediatrician was deemed to be at fault, and the adequacy of the autopsy was also criticised.

Sub-optimal care by obstetricians

It was judged that sub-optimal care by obstetricians might have contributed to five cases of SIDS and to two explained deaths. In three cases, the obstetrician was held partly responsible for the vulnerability of a baby who later died from SIDS: one was the product of a multiple pregnancy induced in a young mother, another was born after unchecked premature labour, and the third was asphyxiated during breech delivery. In another instance, traumatic delivery was thought to have adversely affected a mother's attitude to her baby. Obstetricians were also criticised for poor communication, once with a mother and once with a paediatric colleague, for not heeding a family history of infant deaths, and for poor technique in resuscitating a baby.

EXAMPLE 6

A mother who disliked hospitals ruptured her membranes early and was febrile by the time of delivery. A precautionary culture of the baby's blood grew *Streptococcus pyogenes* group B, and treatment with intravenous antibiotics was started. However, after 48 hours the mother insisted on taking him home and was required to sign a form acknowledging that she was doing so against medical advice. The baby became unwell over the next few days and the general practitioner visited twice, but he had not been informed of the infection. The baby steadily deteriorated and died, and at autopsy was found to have streptococcal pneumonia.

In addition to noting the mother's disregard of medical advice, the panel also criticised the paediatrician for failing to ensure adequate treatment of the baby's infection, and for failing to alert the general practitioner to a potentially dangerous situation.

Sub-optimal care by midwives

Panels criticised hospital midwives in four cases; in two for giving bad advice, in one for not paying enough attention to a mother's psychiatric problems, and in another for failing to recognise a risk of abuse. Community midwives were criticised in nine instances in seven cases: in three for not providing adequate supervision, in two for not recognising the vulnerability of the baby, in two for not making a medical referral for a baby who was unwell, in one for failure to weigh a baby who was feeding poorly, and in one for poor communication.

Sub-optimal care by casualty doctors or nurses

Sub-optimal care by casualty staff was thought possibly to have contributed to five deaths. Casualty doctors were criticised three times, and a casualty nurse once, for failing to get a paediatrician to see a baby that a worried mother had brought to their department. In another instance, the casualty doctor's attempt to resuscitate a baby was thought to be inadequate.

Sub-optimal care by other health professionals

Children's nurses were criticised in two cases on three grounds: failure to recognise significant deterioration in a sick baby, incompetent use of a monitor and poor technique in resuscitation. There was one criticism each of a physiotherapist, for advising a mother whose baby's hips had been unstable to lie him prone, of a specialist nurse, visiting under the scheme for the care of the next infant (CONI), for failing to recognise a risk of abuse, and of an ambulance man, for using the wrong technique in attempting to resuscitate a collapsed baby.

Sub-optimal care by social workers

In evaluating this section, it should be borne in mind that panel membership did not include a social worker, and that if it had the number and nature of the comments might well have been different. As it was, panels thought that sub-optimal care by social workers may have contributed to 21 (6%) of the cases of SIDS (Table 5.6). This proportion reflects the greater incidence of SIDS among disadvantaged families who need social work support and the difficulties that sometimes arise in distinguishing between SIDS and deaths resulting from maltreatment. Statutory responsibility for child protection is vested primarily with social service departments, and the most frequent area of criticism was failure to recognise or act upon a risk of abuse. This usually occurred in cases where the panel suspected that death had arisen from some form of maltreatment, and where a social services department knew about the family but had not taken appropriate preventative measures, such as holding a multidisciplinary conference to agree a plan of protection. Social workers were also criticised for their inadequate support of two disadvantaged mothers who could not cope with their babies, and for allowing inappropriate arrangements for the alternative care of three other babies. Poor communication with the health visitor was also cited on one occasion.

Table 5.6 Sub-optimal care by social workers

Area of concern	Instances	
	n	*%*
Failure to recognise or act upon risk of abuse	15	4.3
Inadequate support for disadvantaged mother	2	0.6
Inappropriate alternative care arrangements for baby	3	0.9
Poor communication with health visitor	1	0.3
Total	21	6.1

EXAMPLE 7

A fourth baby, a girl, was born to a family well known to the social services department. One of their previous children had died suddenly at the age of three months, and the other two were on the Child Protection Register. The health visitor was very concerned about standards of care and visited frequently. On two occasions, the parents said that they had had to shake the baby because she looked pale. One morning at the age of seven weeks she was found dead in her cot. The autopsy showed no evidence of trauma and the death was registered as SIDS.

The panel thought the baby probably died as a result of poor care or maltreatment, and criticised the social worker concerned for failing to convene a multidisciplinary conference at which a plan of supervision and protection could be agreed before the baby left the maternity unit.

Contributory factors involving carers

For deaths that occur at home, it is to be expected that the behaviour of parents and other carers should come under careful scrutiny. In 187 cases (54%) of SIDS, panels identified a total of 397 factors involving parents or other carers that they thought might have contributed to the death. In many cases, more than one member of the family was implicated. Panels also noted 54 factors relating to carers in 24 (34%) of the explained deaths. The people involved are shown in Table 5.7. As would be expected, mothers, with or without their partners, were the carers most frequently involved. The relatively small number of criticisms specific to fathers reflects the infrequency with which fathers look after babies on their own. Grandparents and other relatives were sometimes involved, but there was only one instance involving a baby minder outside the family.

Table 5.7 Carers involved in contributory factors

Carer	SIDS		Explained deaths	
	n = 346	%	n = 71	%
Both parents	117	33.8	14	19.7
Mother	89	25.7	9	12.7
Father	20	5.8	0	0
Grandparents	13	3.8	1	1.4
Other relatives	3	0.9	0	0
Baby minder	1	0.3	0	0
Total of cases involving carers	187 *	54.0	24	33.8

* Many cases involved more than one carer

Table 5.8 gives details of all the contributory factors involving carers that were identified. Some of these could be described as sub-optimal care for which the person concerned could fairly be held responsible, but others were circumstances, such as poverty or depression, over which he or she could have little or no control. In many cases, several different factors were noted.

The factors are listed under under six different headings: personal situation, social circumstances, substance abuse, infant care, sleeping arrangements and use of services.

The areas incurring most frequent criticism were substance abuse and sleeping arrangements. Variation between panels was apparent here, with some but not all panels identifying as a contributory factor anything known to be associated with an increased risk of SIDS, such as smoking or prone sleeping. A more objective assessment of the prevalence and significance of these factors can be made from the case-control study.

Personal and social circumstances

Most of the aspects of the mother's personal situation that panels thought might possibly have contributed to the death of her baby, such as depression and lack of support, were factors for which she could not be held responsible. Social circumstances were also thought to have played a part in several deaths, in particular when the family was oppressed by poverty, or followed a chaotic life style.

Substance abuse

Smoking, identified in previous studies as conferring an increased risk of SIDS, was noted by panels in 100 instances, much more than for any other factor. Use of illegal drugs was cited 24 times, and excessive consumption of alcohol 13 times. Several parents were criticised for abuse of all three types of substance. In addition, 13 carers were held to be possibly responsible for the death when they had been looking after the baby while under the influence of alcohol.

Table 5.8 Contibutory factors involving carers

Area of concern	Instances			
	SIDS		Explained deaths	
	n = 346	%	n = 71	%
Personal situation (total)	*26*	*7.5*	*6*	*8.5*
Maternal depression	6	1.7	1	1.4
Other illness in mother	2	0.6	0	0
Poor hygiene	4	1.2	0	0
Poor bonding	3	0.9	0	0
Lack of support	5	1.4	1	1.4
Immaturity of mother	1	0.3	1	1.4
Learning difficulties of mother	1	0.3	0	0
Violence of father	0	0	1	1.4
Mendacity	1	0.3	0	0
Prostitution	1	0.3	0	0
Poor command of English	0	0	1	1.4
Mother absent from home	0	0	1	1.4
Mother abused in childhood	2	0.6	0	0
Social circumstances (total)	*21*	*6.1*	*3*	*4.2*
Poverty	8	2.3	2	2.8
Disorganised household	10	2.9	0	0
Travelling family	1	0.3	1	1.4
Mother in prison	1	0.3	0	0
Father in prison	1	0.3	0	0
Substance abuse (total)	*137*	*39.6*	*14*	*19.7*
Cigarettes	100	28.9	8	11.3
Alcohol	13	3.8	4	5.6
Illegal drugs	24	6.9	2	2.8
Infant care (total)	*45*	*13.0*	*7*	*9.9*
Incorrect feeding	7	2.0	2	2.8
Inadequate supervision of baby	7	2.0	4	5.6
Suspected abuse	8	2.3	0	0
Carer under influence of alcohol	13	3.8	0	0
Generally poor standards	10	2.9	1	1.4
Sleeping arrangements (total)	*137*	*39.6*	*6*	*8.5*
Inappropriate place	12	3.5	0	0
Use of unsafe cot or bunk-bed	0	0	3	4.2
Settee shared with adult	6	1.7	0	0
Bed-sharing under influence of alcohol	13	3.8	0	0
Other bed-sharing	19	5.5	1	1.4

Table 5.8 Contibutory factors involving carers *cont.*

Area of concern	Instances			
	SIDS		Explained deaths	
	n = 346	%	n = 71	%
Use of soft pillow	5	1.4	0	0
Placing baby prone	31	9.0	1	1.4
Overwrapping	29	8.4	0	0
Keeping baby too warm	16	4.6	1	1.4
Use of electric blanket	1	0.3	0	0
Leaving fire burning near baby all night	4	1.2	0	0
Not keeping baby warm enough	1	0.3	0	0
Use of services (total)	*31*	*9.0*	*15*	*21.1*
Late booking at antenatal clinic	5	1.4	2	2.8
Refusal to use services or accept advice	15	4.3	2	2.8
Failure to give medication or other treatment	2	0.6	1	1.4
Failure to recognise illness or seek advice	8	2.3	7	9.9
Refusal of hospital admission for baby	0	0	1	1.4
Taking baby out of hospital against advice	0	0	1	1.4
Incorrect resuscitation	1	0.3	1	1.4

EXAMPLE 8

A 30-year-old mother looked after her four children without support, her partner having left her soon after the birth of the youngest. She was on treatment for chronic arthritis, anxiety and depression, and was prone to the abuse of alcohol and other drugs. Her flat was burgled, so she went to stay with her mother, with whom she had a stormy relationship, in very cramped accommodation. The two women smoked a total of about 40 cigarettes a day. Her fourth baby, a boy, had been asphyxiated at birth and was slow in his development. When three months old, he became unwell and would not feed, and was found dead in his cot in the early evening. No abnormalities were found at autopsy and the death was registered as SIDS.

The panel thought that the multiplicity of problems besetting this mother must have contributed to the death of her baby.

Infant care and sleeping arrangements

Other areas of poor infant care were inadequate supervision and incorrect feeding, usually the introduction of solids too early. In eight cases of SIDS child abuse was raised as a possible contributory factor. This difficult issue is discussed in the section 'Deaths resulting from maltreatment' below. With regard to sleeping arrangements, the commonest criticisms were laying the baby prone (31 instances) and overwrapping (28 instances), both of which recent studies had shown to bring an increased risk of SIDS. There were also 16 criticisms for keeping the baby too warm, in contrast to only one for not keeping him or her warm enough. Panels varied in their judgements on bed-sharing, reflecting current uncertainties on the issue. Sharing a bed with an intoxicated adult, or sleeping together on a settee, were usually regarded as hazardous, being cited in 13 and six cases respectively, while bed-sharing in the absence of these particular hazards was thought to be a possible contributory factor in 19 other cases. Other places regarded as inappropriate for a baby to sleep were the floor, on sofas, on full-sized beds, or in car seats. It is a tragic irony that at least three parents had transferred their babies to such places because of the publicity given to the alleged risk from cot mattresses, later shown to be unfounded [3]. Two of the explained deaths arose when a baby was accidentally hung after slipping under the horizontal bar of a bunk-bed designed for an older child, and a third baby died when a faulty cot collapsed. Parents were criticised on five occasions for leaving their baby to sleep close to coke or gas fires. Soft pillows and an electric blanket were also seen as potential sources of danger.

EXAMPLE 9

A boy aged three months had oral thrush, a nappy rash and a mild respiratory infection for which he was taking antibiotics. His parents went out to a party leaving him in the care of a babysitter. They came home just after midnight, having drunk a lot of alcohol, and put the baby down to sleep in his cot beside their bed as usual. They woke at 8.00 a.m. to find the baby dead, lying in their bed and totally covered by the duvet. They could not remember what had happened during the night, but thought they had probably taken the baby into their bed for a feed and then fallen asleep. No significant abnormalities were found at autopsy and the death was registered as SIDS.

The panel thought that the baby's death resulted from sharing a bed with parents who were intoxicated.

EXAMPLE 10

A six-month-old boy with a history of wheezing became chesty and unwell. Both parents used to smoke constantly in the presence of the baby, despite advice from the health visitor. The mother was depressed, and the father, who was unemployed, took most of the decisions and was adverse to anyone in authority. The general practitioner came to see the baby and advised admission to hospital. This was refused, as was another attempt at persuasion by the health visitor when she called later. Next morning, the baby was found dead in his cot. The autopsy showed extensive bronchiolitis and pneumonia.

The panel thought that the death might have been avoided if the parents had not refused to allow the baby to go into hospital. In addition, their heavy smoking was thought to have contributed to the illness.

Use of services

Several families were criticised for an apparent aversion to seeking or taking advice about the health of their babies. The most extreme instances were a mother who insisted on taking her baby out of hospital when he was in the early stages of an infection that proved fatal, and a father who refused to let his sick baby be admitted for hospital care. In seven cases very late booking for antenatal care was thought to have contributed to subsequent death. In eight cases of SIDS and seven of explained death, panels thought that parents had failed to appreciate the severity of their baby's illness and had not sought vital help. In three other instances, parents did seek advice but then failed to give the treatment prescribed.

EXAMPLE 11

A girl born seven weeks prematurely made good progress while in hospital, but the health visitor found it difficult to obtain access to see her once she had gone home. One morning when she was four months old, her grandmother found her seriously ill and took her straight to hospital, but she died a few hours later. The story emerged that she had been unwell for three days, crying incessantly and feeding poorly. She then became very hot and drowsy. When her grandmother happened to call, she found the baby unresponsive, with wandering eyes and stiff limbs. The parents said they had not contacted the doctor because they disliked his manner.

Autopsy revealed cerebral oedema and encephalopathy, thought to be of viral origin. The panel concluded that this baby might not have died if the parents had made proper use of the services.

Carers other than mothers

Fathers and other relatives were criticised for much the same reasons as were mothers. In addition, three fathers were thought to have contributed to the death of a baby by their failure to support their partner, and two grandparents by damaging their daughter's capacity as a mother through their abuse of her as a child. The one criticism of a baby minder was for failure to provide adequate supervision.

Inadequate resources

Panels identified 14 instances in which inadequate resources were thought to have contributed to SIDS, but only one instance involving an explained death (Table 5.9). Ten related to the material circumstances of the family, usually the adequacy of accommodation. Of those that related to the health service, there were three criticisms for the absence of cover for a health visitor who was off sick, and two for the lack of facilities for paediatric intensive care. The latter deficiency has since been officially acknowledged and is being addressed on a national basis.

Table 5.9 Inadequate resources

Resource	SIDS		Explained deaths	
	n = 346	%	*n = 71*	%
Poor accommodation	9	2.6	0	0
Poor heating	1	0.3	0	0
Lack of cover for health visitor	3	0.9	0	0
Lack of facilities for paediatric intensive care	1	0.3	1	1.4
Total of cases involving carers	14	4.0	1	1.4

DEATHS RESULTING FROM MALTREATMENT

Panel assessment

As well as identifying instances of sub-optimal care, panels were required to place each death in one of several broad clinico-pathological categories [4,5]. One of these categories was for cases in which maltreatment by carers was considered to be a major factor contributing to the death. Maltreatment was taken to cover a wide spectrum ranging from deliberate action, such as smothering, to negligence and extremely poor care. In making this assessment, panels were guided by published descriptions of deaths caused by covert maltreatment [6–10]. From these reports, features giving rise for concern might include: in the family, a previous unexplained infant death or non-accidental injuries; in a parent, a history of abuse as a child, followed by personality disorder and self-harm; in the baby, previous injuries or episodes of sudden illness, such as apnoeic attacks, that were inadequately explained; such episodes all occurring in the presence of the same carer; and a death outside the usual age range for SIDS. These characteristics have been confirmed, with additional features, in a recent more extensive report by Meadow [11]. In the light of such guidance, the panels carefully scrutinised all the circumstances and all the available records for each case, seeking to arrive at a balanced collective judgement. Nevertheless, because the evidence was never more than circumstantial, the conclusions reached were always ultimately subjective.

Panels' conclusions on maltreatment

Table 5.10 sets out the number of cases in each of the two categories in which panels thought that maltreatment might have played a part. Among the 346 cases of SIDS that they examined, panels concluded that maltreatment was probably the main cause of death in 22 (6%), and a secondary or alternative cause in a further 28 (8%). Maltreatment was also thought to have contributed to some of the 71 explained deaths, but a smaller proportion than for SIDS, being cited as the main cause of death in three and as an alternative or secondary cause in four. Thus, overall there was a concern about maltreatment in 14% of SIDS and in 10% of explained deaths.

EXAMPLE 1

A six-week-old baby boy was treated in a casualty department for a fractured femur, said to have been caused by falling off his mother's bed. The casualty nurse noted that the mother, who now had a new partner, seemed rather detached from the baby, and she alerted the general practitioner and health visitor. A week later, the mother asked the general practitioner to send the baby to hospital because of a minor respiratory infection, but he thought admission was unnecessary and treated with antibiotics at home. Two weeks later, while in his mother's care, the baby was found dead in his cot in the early afternoon with a soft toy over his face. No abnormality was found at autopsy, there was no police investigation and the death was registered as SIDS.

The panel thought that this baby's fracture probably resulted from maltreatment, and that the same was probably also true of his death.

Table 5.10 Cases in which panels suspected maltreatment

	SIDS		Explained deaths		All SUDI	
	n = 346	%	n = 71	%	n = 417	%
Maltreatment thought to be main cause of death	22	6.4	3	4.2	25	6.0
Maltreatment thought to be secondary or alternative cause of death	28	8.1	4	5.6	32	7.7
Total in which possibility of maltreatment was cited	50	14.5	7	9.9	57	13.7

EXAMPLE 2

The parents had lost a previous child at the age of eight months, the death being attributed to SIDS. Their new baby, a girl, seemed normal and healthy at birth, but from the age of six weeks the mother reported a series of unusual attacks during which the baby went stiff and turned blue. On each occasion, the general practitioner was called but found nothing wrong, and no one else witnessed an attack. Finally, at the age of five months, the baby was found dead in her cot after a restless night when her mother had got up to her twice because of her crying. The autopsy included full metabolic studies but found no significant abnormality and the death was registered as SIDS.

The panel allocated this death to the category in which there was no evidence of any illness, citing the category of maltreatment as an alternative on the suspicion that the baby might have been subjected to recurrent suffocation.

EXAMPLE 3

A 16-year-old single mother who regularly used cannabis was looking after her niece aged 18 months as well as her seven-month-old son. While she was bathing them together, she went to answer the telephone, and on finishing a quite lengthy conversation came back to find the smaller baby submerged in the bath water and dead.

The autopsy established that death was caused by drowning, which was registered as accidental. However, the panel concluded that the supervision of this baby had been so negligent that the death should be listed among those for which maltreatment was a secondary cause.

Cases undergoing police investigation

The protocol for the study excluded from confidential enquiry cases in which there was an early suspicion of non-accidental injury leading to ongoing investigation by the police (see section 'Excluded data', Chapter 2). Fourteen such cases were identified, most of which led to criminal prosecution. Comparison with Office of National Statistics (ONS) figures revealed eight further deaths in the relevant period and areas that were not notified to the study, and it is known that at least six of these were subject to police investigation. Overall, therefore, during the course of the study the police carried out ongoing investigations into at least 20 and possibly 22 cases, none of which were presented for confidential enquiry.

Total sudden deaths in which maltreatment was suspected

The total number of sudden unexpected deaths in the study areas was 464, which includes eight not notified to the study and 39 notified but not taken to confidential enquiry (Chapter 3) in addition to the 417 that came before panels. If those subject to police investigation are added to those identified by panels, there was a suggestion that some form of maltreatment might have contributed to between 77 and 79 cases (17%), the evidence ranging in strength from that sufficient to justify criminal prosecution to that giving rise to the suspicion of an expert group. This proportion is close to that found in a national survey of coroners' post-mortems carried out for three months in 1995, which included 84 sudden infant deaths. Coroners stated that they initially regarded 15 of these deaths (18%) as suspicious [12].

Published figures for homicide in infancy

Figures for recognised homicide, where the cause of death has been established by the coroner and may have led to criminal prosecution, can be derived from the ONS or from Home Office statistics. The ONS lists deaths in infants aged between one and 12 months under two relevant headings in the ninth revision of the International Classification of Diseases (ICD): code E 960–969, which covers various forms of homicide, and E 980–989, which lists deaths resulting from 'injury undetermined whether accidentally or purposely afflicted' [13]. Deaths may be placed in the latter category pending a coroner's verdict, and most are eventually reassigned to the heading of homicide [14]. Combining these two ICD groups gives totals of 24 deaths in 1997, 26 in 1996, 15 in 1995, 24 in 1994 and 29 in 1993. Home Office criminal statistics show a relatively constant rate for homicide in infancy (including the first month) of around 30 deaths per year [15]. The number of cases subject to ongoing police investigation during the SUDI study is broadly in line with these figures. It is recognised that a person in England and Wales is four times more likely to be the victim of homicide in the first year of life than at any subsequent age [15].

Deaths resulting from unrecognised maltreatment

In addition to these deaths in which homicide is recognised, it has long been thought likely that covert maltreatment may sometimes play a part in other unexpected deaths in infancy that have been officially attributed to cot death or other causes. This is an area of much uncertainty and imprecision, and it is not possible to be sure of the numbers involved. Parents who kill their babies usually do so alone and in secret and seldom afterwards admit what has really happened. They may not have intended to kill, but may have acted for various other reasons, such as exasperation and loss of control, the wish to stop the baby's crying, extreme carelessness, or sometimes the need to gain attention for themselves. Other members of the family may have no suspicions, or if they do may not voice them. The most thorough autopsy cannot distinguish between death from natural causes and death caused by suffocation. If the death is attributed to SIDS, it is understandable that the attention of all those dealing with the family should be mainly directed to the provision of sympathy and support. Occasionally, the true cause of death may eventually come to light, for example when a parent makes a later confession or is observed by means of covert video surveillance in the act of harming another baby [16]. Usually, however, there is never any firm evidence, and the true number of unexpected deaths that result from maltreatment can only be a matter of conjecture.

Previous estimates of the scale of the problem

There have been few previous assessments of the number of infant deaths that result from unrecognised homicide. From 1976 to 1979, a study of 988 deaths between the ages of one week and two years was conducted in eight large urban areas in England and Scotland (Multicentre Study) [17]. In addition to nine deaths officially certified as homicide, case conferences thought that a further 15 deaths certified as accidental might also have in fact resulted from homicide. However, maltreatment was not mentioned as a possible cause in any of the 293 deaths registered as SIDS – although in some instances the reliability of the account given by parents was questioned.

In 1985, Emery suggested that among deaths classified as SIDS between 2% and 10%, varying from place to place, might in fact result from what he termed filicide [18]. Confidential enquiries into 115 sudden unexpected post-perinatal deaths occurring in Sheffield between 1980 and 1988 identified parental action as a major factor in eight (7%) [4]. In Scotland and Avon, however, the proportion was thought to be smaller [19,20]. On the assumption that the rate for deaths arising from maltreatment remains more or less constant, the proportion that applied in the 1980s would be considerably greater today, when the total of unexpected deaths has fallen. After adjustment for this, the number of deaths that the SUDI panels attributed to maltreatment lies towards the lower end of the range suggested by Emery. In addition, some of the difference between the estimates of earlier and later studies may reflect a developing awareness of the problem.

Difficulties in dealing with unexpected deaths in infancy

Awareness that maltreatment may sometimes be involved creates great difficulties for all those who encounter a sudden death in infancy – family, friends and voluntary agencies as well as doctors, health visitors, social workers, pathologists, coroners and their officers, and the police. The majority of families whose baby dies unexpectedly, probably at least four out of five, are innocent of blame and have suffered one of the most grievous blows that fate can inflict. Their need is for sympathy and support, backed up by expert advice and counselling. Insensitive interrogation and ill-concealed suspicion of abuse will cruelly compound their grief. On the other hand, it is important to try and identify the minority of cases in which a carer has caused the death, so that appropriate interventions can be made with those involved, and so that other children, particularly those as yet unborn, can be protected. Many instances are known in which parents have brought about the death of two or more successive babies before the cause was recognised [7,10,11,21].

Investigation of sudden infant deaths

Striking the right balance between sympathy and dispassionate assessment presents professionals with an extremely difficult task. It is essential that those who have to deal with a newly bereaved family should be well-informed and experienced, as well as sensitive and understanding. The role of the coroner's officer can be crucial: his or her initial report may often determine whether there is a police investigation and guide the coroner in the choice of pathologist, thereby setting the direction and tone of subsequent management. In addition, this report is frequently the only information available to the pathologist when he or she has to decide which features to look for in the autopsy. Yet the report has to be completed in haste, so that autopsy and funeral are not delayed, and there is seldom the opportunity to carry out all the consultation with those who know the family and all the research into previous history needed to help identify possible causes of death, both natural and suspicious.

The report of the coroner's officer, or the pathologist's transcription of it, was usually included in the documents put before the panels in the SUDI study. Frequently, the information given was thought to be inadequate. It was suggested that reports would be improved if the coroner's officer routinely consulted a paediatrician with an interest in infant death or, failing this, followed a checklist of points that should be covered [22]. It is an anomaly that when a baby is sick a doctor expects to have a full history before making a diagnosis, but when a baby has died the pathologist may be expected to do without an adequate history and make a diagnosis by examination alone. This anomaly is accentuated by the conclusion of the pathologists in the SUDI study that the single most useful component of the investigation is a very detailed clinical history (see Chapter 4).

The autopsy following unexpected infant deaths

If the pathologist is not briefed as fully as possible he or she may not carry out all the relevant investigations, and the unique opportunity afforded by the autopsy may be wasted. It is a serious disservice to the bereaved family if, for example, inherited metabolic disease goes undetected at autopsy because the pathologist has not been told of a history that would result in the appropriate tests. Similarly, ignorance of previous suspicion of abuse might result in the omission of a skeletal survey at autopsy and the failure to detect maltreatment as the probable cause of death.

In some areas, it appears that coroners, perhaps concerned about the proportion of deaths thought to result from maltreatment, are routinely instructing a forensic pathologist to do the autopsy after any sudden unexpected death in infancy. The findings from the pathology component of the SUDI study (Chapter 4) suggest that this practice has an important disadvantage. While they are skilled at detecting evidence of unnatural death, once this has been excluded forensic pathologists are less likely than their paediatric colleagues to carry out the detailed microbiological, metabolic and histological studies that may reveal the diagnosis in a death from natural causes. This may in part result from the regulations that govern payment for ancillary tests in autopsies ordered by coroners. The Third Annual Report for CESDI recommended that autopsies on infants dying suddenly and unexpectedly should, wherever possible, be carried out by a paediatric pathologist, or a general pathologist with a special interest, working in conjunction with a forensic pathologist if the coroner so wishes [23]. Such an arrangement is already working well in some areas, and as the number of infant deaths falls and the number of specialist pathologists increases this ideal should become achievable throughout the country. Experience has shown that referring infant autopsies to a specialist unit need not cause delays if sufficient priority is given. Occasional paediatric practice should be regarded as unacceptable for pathology as it is for surgery.

Importance of local case discussion

Sometimes the complete picture of an unexpected death will only become clear when all those concerned have been able to contribute their piece of the jigsaw. This was one of the main reasons for the recommendation that a local case discussion should be held after every sudden unexpected death in infancy [24]. The procedure for such discussions is described in the section 'Local case discussion', Chapter 2. They are best held as soon as the full autopsy results become available, and essential participants include the family doctor and the health visitor, as well as the pathologist and a paediatrician with a special interest in the subject. Meadow maintains that the present arrangements for the investigation of sudden unexpected deaths in infancy are unsatisfactory and in need of revision [11]. Some of the findings of the SUDI study would appear to support his contention, and the recommendations arising from the study include proposals for an improved system (see Chapter 7, 'Investigation and procedures following sudden unexpected deaths in infancy').

Prevention of deaths arising from maltreatment

Human nature being what it is, there is little prospect that deaths from maltreatment can be totally eliminated. However, some benefit might be achieved by better targeting of surveillance and support from health and social workers to those families who are at greatest risk. Since the risk factors for child abuse are similar to those for unexpected infant deaths in general, targeting would cover a high proportion of babies who are vulnerable in either respect. It would help health visitors and social workers in this task if there were better ways of identifying families who are at risk, just as it would help pathologists if there were better ways of distinguishing between natural and unnatural deaths. More research is needed in both these areas. With this in mind, it is planned that data from the SUDI study should be used to compare the epidemiological and pathological features of deaths that the panels thought were suspicious with deaths that were thought to be innocent. However, whatever advances are made in our understanding of sudden infant deaths, it is likely that some degree of uncertainty will always cloud the issue of those that result from maltreatment.

References

1. Department of Health. *Confidential Enquiry into Stillbirths and Deaths in Infancy: Third Annual Report*. London: DoH, 1996: chapter 7.

2. Department of Health. *Confidential Enquiry into Stillbirths and Deaths in Infancy: Second Annual Report*. London: DoH, 1995: para 5.5.

3. Department of Health. *The Report of the Expert Group to Investigate Cot Death Theories: Toxic Gas Hypothesis* (Limerick report). London: DoH, 1998.

4. Taylor, EM and Emery, JL. 'Categories of preventable unexpected infant deaths', *Archives of Diseases in Childhood*, 1990; 65: 535–9.

5. Department of Health. *Confidential Enquiry into Stillbirths and Deaths in Infancy: Third Annual Report*. London: DoH, 1996: para 7.3.1.

6. Meadow, R. 'Suffocation, recurrent apnoea and sudden infant death', *Journal of Pediatrics*, 1990; 117: 351–7.

7. Emery, JL. 'Child abuse, sudden infant death syndrome, and unexpected infant death', *Am. J. Dis. Child.*, 1993; 147: 1097–1100.

8. British Paediatric Association. *Evaluation of suspected imposed upper airway obstruction*, report of working party. London: BPA, 1994.

9. American Academy of Pediatrics. 'Distinguishing sudden infant death syndrome from child abuse fatalities', *Pediatrics*, 1994; 94: 124–6.

10. Reece, RM. 'Fatal child abuse and sudden infant death syndrome: a critical diagnostic decision', *Pediatrics*, 1993; 91: 423–9.

11. Meadow, R. 'Unnatural sudden infant death', *Archives of Diseases in Childhood*, 1999; 80: 7–14.

12. Office for National Statistics: Social Survey Division. *Coroners' post mortems in England and Wales: a report for the Department of Health*. London: ONS 1997: table 5.4a.

13. Office for National Statistics. *Mortality statistics: childhood, infant and perinatal, England and Wales*. London: ONS, 1992–6: series DH3.

14. Office for National Statistics. *Mortality statistics: childhood, infant and perinatal, England and Wales*. London: ONS, 1996: series DH3, chap 2, xix.

15. Marks, MN and Kumar, R. 'Infanticide in England and Wales', *Med. Sci. Law*, 1993; 33: 329–39.

16. Samuels, MP, McClaughlin, W, Jacobson, RR, Poets, CF and Southall, DP. 'Fourteen cases of imposed upper airway obstruction', *Archives of Diseases in Childhood*, 1992; 67: 162–70.

17. Knowelden, J, Keeling, J, Nicoll, JP. *A Multicentre Study of Post-neonatal Mortality*. University of Sheffield: Medical Care Research Unit, 1984.

18. Emery, JL. 'Infanticide, filicide and cot death', *Archives of Diseases in Childhood*, 1985; 60: 505–7.

19. Arneil, GC, Gibson, AAM, McIntosh, H, Brooke, H, Harvie, A and Patrick, WJA. 'National post-perinatal infant mortality and cot death study, Scotland 1981–82', *Lancet*, 1985; i: 740–3.

20. Fleming, PJ, Berry, PJ, Gilbert, R, Golding, J, Rudd, PT, Hall, E, White, D and Holton, J. 'Categories of preventable sudden unexpected infant deaths' (letter), *Archives of Diseases in Childhood*, 1991; 66: 170–1.

21. Wolkind, S, Taylor, EM, Waite, AJ, Dalton, M and Emery, JL. 'Recurrence of unexpected infant death', *Act. Paed.*, 1993; 82: 873–6.

22. Department of Health. *Confidential Enquiry into Stillbirths and Deaths in Infancy: Third Annual Report*. London: DoH, 1996: para 9.5.1.

23. Ibid: para 9.4.5.

24. Ibid: para 9.3.9.

Chapter 6

The Perspective of the Research Interviewers

Pam Mueller and Shirley Stephenson

Preface

Interviewing bereaved parents challenges you personally as well as professionally. It is not possible to remain a detached observer because your own feelings about children and death are inevitably drawn in. The experience of each interviewer in the SUDI study will therefore be personally unique, but we hope that this account is a fair representation.

Background of interviewers

All of us had previously served as health visitors or community midwives in a primary health care team, which proved an excellent preparation for the role of interviewer for several reasons. Firstly, we were readily accepted by all members of the primary health care teams we encountered; we had practical knowledge and experience of community health, and were sensitive to the extra demand we would be making on busy health professionals. Secondly, as health visitors or midwives we were used to functioning independently, to visiting homes of all sorts, and to responding to unpredictable family crises, including bereavement. Thirdly, we were accustomed to knocking on the doors of strangers and accepting any problem or emotion that might be there to greet us. Most of a health visitor's work takes place in other people's homes – their territory, not ours – and a non-judgmental and respectful approach is essential. We believe that no other discipline would have been as well prepared for the task of interviewer as health visitors.

In order to enhance our communication skills, some of us undertook training in counselling during the course of the study. The supervision by an experienced colleague that formed part of this training proved particularly helpful. If circumstances had allowed, it would have been valuable if a similar form of professional supervision could have been provided for all interviewers from the outset of the study.

Although health visitors and midwives are often required to collect data for the purposes of audit, few of us had previous experience of formal research. Knowledge and skills in research, after a modicum of training, had to be learned along the way. The eight original interviewers stayed with the study throughout its duration, building up an invaluable informal network of support. Those of our colleagues who were appointed on a temporary short-term basis were not as fortunate, being frustrated by the lack of continuity and by the inability to build confidence from experience.

Training

The study began on 1 February 1993. We were appointed in December 1992 and met together for the first time the following month, so we had a great deal to learn and plan in a very short space of time. The questionnaire was already in draft form and we were immediately involved in the processes of piloting and amending. Training sessions were arranged with the study's statistician, with the aim of ensuring consistency in the application of the questionnaire and avoidance of interviewer bias. The time available for piloting the questionnaire with volunteer families was very short, and we would have felt more confident if we had been more familiar with the document by the time the study began.

Throughout the study, there were regular liaison meetings, where practice could be updated and experiences shared. New interviewers were included as soon as they joined the team, so that they could learn from the accumulating experience of their colleagues. Peer support was a vital element for us, and since we worked so far apart there was much informal contact by telephone.

Dealing with bereavement

Initially, we spent two days as a group having formal teaching about bereavement. This was extremely beneficial, although perhaps not long enough. We learned about the range of normal grief reactions, and how our own beliefs about death might influence our responses and affect the families we dealt with. This part of our training helped to nurture a supportive bond between us. Because of our background in health visiting or midwifery, we required little training in the handling of professionals. However, working alongside professionals who were trying to deal with bereavement in others was a new experience, and we learned that they needed to be treated almost with the same care and sensitivity that was required for the bereaved family. They, too, had a need to be looked after.

Management of data

At the completion of each interview, the data had to be entered into the laptop computer supplied to each researcher. Initially, few of us felt really confident with computers, but after training and practice, inputting data became a straightforward procedure. Regular audit took place to check consistency, particularly in the early stages, and any queries were dealt with by the statistician. At the end of the study, all the researchers were involved in the process of data cleaning, a laborious but vital exercise. The importance of strict coding became more obvious at that stage, and if we had appreciated this from the outset earlier ambiguities might have been reduced.

Feasibility of the protocol

The protocol for the SUDI study was clear and worked well in practice. Modifications were made in the light of experience and after general consultation. The addition of the antimony component raised some practical issues, but these were easily resolved after discussion and practice. Our confidence grew as we saw that our experience and opinions were valued and responded to by the leaders of the research team.

Notification network

Each researcher built upon the system for reporting baby deaths that already operated in his or her area, and a combination of methods for notification were adopted. The district coordinators for CESDI were a good contact, particularly in those areas which already had an effective system for reporting infant deaths. In some areas, however, this system did not prove to be sufficiently rapid and alternative ways had to be considered. Accident and paediatric departments were asked to report all relevant deaths as soon as possible, and were given the number of the researcher's telephone answering machine, specially supplied for this purpose. One case was reported by a conscientious junior doctor at three o'clock in the morning.

Coroners and their officers were also approached in one district, proving to be the most rapid source of notification. A good working relationship with coroner's officers was also helpful when the cause of death was uncertain, since the protocol excluded cases which the police were investigating with a view to possible criminal proceedings.

Various other sources were also used for notification, including paediatricians, clinical medical officers, pathologists and voluntary organisations such as the Foundation for the Study of Infant Deaths (FSID). Although these sources were not as rapid as those mentioned earlier, they helped to ensure that all relevant cases were identified. The advice of the local paediatrician would often guide us in deciding whether or not a more complicated case met the criteria for inclusion in the study.

Introduction to the family

As soon as we learned of a death, usually within 24 hours, we would contact the family's health visitor to discuss the process of the study and the family circumstances. Health visitors had all been made aware of the study through their professional channels, but delays were sometimes encountered when they felt it necessary to seek advice from their manager. Other factors that sometimes led to delays in the initial contact were weekends, bank holidays and annual leave. The health visitor who was familiar to the family usually worked well as a caring route of entry. For babies under two weeks old, whose supervision had not yet been transferred to the health visitor, the introduction was effected by the community midwife. It was unusual for the interviewer to have to go in 'cold' on her own. In order to see families at the earliest opportunity possible for them and their health visitor, we had to work very flexible hours, frequently visiting in evenings or at weekends. The unsettled life style of some families and their inaccessibility by telephone made planning more difficult.

Selection of controls

Control families were identified through the health visitor as previously described in Chapter 2. The process was best managed by going through the birth register together, otherwise there was a tendency for our thoughtful colleagues to weed out families they thought unsuitable for interview, such as those with noisy households or fierce dogs. We had to emphasise that exclusions were only allowed when participation might be harmful for the family. We sometimes encountered difficulties when the health visitor normally responsible for an area was absent, or where there were not enough babies in a case load to provide the requisite number of controls. On several occasions, we had to decline the offers of mothers who volunteered themselves as controls: news of a baby's death travels quickly within a community and local families soon became aware of the SUDI study.

Despite flexible working hours, there were occasionally problems in conducting interviews with control families within the specified time, especially during the summer and school holidays. The busy and unpredictable nature of the work made it very difficult to provide cover for each other's absence on leave. Cases would then involve travelling outside our usual area and would take much longer, putting us under a great deal of pressure. We had to become experts in juggling and in time management, and often needed recourse to our mutual support network.

Dealing with parents

Initially, we were concerned about the acceptability of early visits, feeling personal compassion as well as professional responsibility towards the bereaved families. The last thing we wanted to do was add to their pain and suffering. However, we soon came to believe that an early visit encouraged the family to talk together about their baby's death and to make a start in the grieving that was essential for them. The role of professionals in supporting bereaved parents is quite different from that of their family and friends. Both roles are important, and both need to be carried out from an early stage and with great sensitivity. For many parents, their supportive network of relatives and neighbours was also grieving, and they felt inhibited from talking about the baby's death as much as they wanted because it caused too much pain for everybody. We soon came to realise that early professional contact was beneficial not only for the accuracy of the study but also for the support of the parents. We provided a listening ear, giving them permission to go over and over the events surrounding the baby's death as they tried to make some sense of it and accept its reality. We believe that the opportunity we gave them to express this natural urge was therapeutic.

Responses to the death of a baby may vary and we had no prior relationship that might enable us to anticipate them, so we approached the first meeting without preconceptions in an unstructured and parent-centred way. We encouraged parents to talk about what they wished, in their own manner and at their own pace, and we accepted without judgement whatever they chose to tell us. We did not take notes while they were speaking, but before leaving we asked if we could write down what they had told us.

If, after an explanation of the study, the family did not wish to participate, we did not press them but invited them to contact us later if they changed their minds, which they sometimes did up to several weeks later. Parents whose baby had a pre-existing problem or had died from a specific condition were, understandably, less likely to see the relevance of the study. There was particular difficulty if one parent was in favour of participation while the other was against; we were aware how much they needed each other's support at this time and we had no wish to come between them. More often, families were eager to do anything they could to help prevent a similar tragedy befalling others, saying that participation in the study seemed one positive contribution when everything else was so negative. Sometimes parents almost seemed to hope that participation would give them the answer to the all-consuming question of why their baby had died; the inevitability of disappointing them made us all the more aware of their courage.

After we had established a rapport at the first meeting, a second visit was seldom refused. The questionnaire, a rather formidable booklet containing 600 items, was not produced until this second visit, which usually did not take place until after the funeral had been held. The questionnaire took about two hours to complete, longer if things had to be taken slowly or if small children were around. We stressed that all information would be anonymised, so as to encourage more honest answers. Sitting beside the parents, we went through each item in the questionnaire, carefully explaining its meaning and purpose. Most of the time, we sensed that the answers we were given were full and honest. The family health visitor was not invited to this second interview in order to encourage the parents to be open and have trust in confidentiality. If any issues arose that we felt could be helpfully shared with the health visitor, we would say so at the end of the meeting but left the parents to pursue this themselves. Before departing, we gave names and telephone numbers of possible contacts, and if the parents so wished we gave information about bereavement, finding the FSID leaflets particularly suitable. We did not attempt to provide ongoing support ourselves. No matter how much we might have wanted to, we were in no position to do so, and we were quite clear that that the family health visitor was the most appropriate contact for long-term support.

After discussions with many parents and various health workers, it became apparent that there were wide variations between professionals in their perceptions of the needs of bereaved families and in the support they provided. In an attempt to quantify these variations, questions about bereavement support were added to the questionnaire.

Dealings with professionals

The support we received from family health visitors was generally very positive and enthusiastic, and without it we could not have achieved such a high consent rate. A few health visitors were resistant to early visits to bereaved families, believing them to be potentially harmful, whereas our experience showed the opposite to be the case. Occasionally, the health visitor's reluctance to introduce us meant that our first contact with the family had to be by telephone, which was far less satisfactory and only used as a last resort. We had to remind ourselves that this might be the first time the health visitor had been involved in the death of a baby and that she too might be in need of support. Sometimes we felt that we had to support the professionals so that they in turn could support the family. It was particularly difficult for a doctor or health visitor if they had seen the baby a day or two prior to the death. Often they felt they must have missed something and that the family would hold this against them. Many health visitors who at first had reservations about the study later commented how beneficial their involvement in it had proved to their subsequent relationship with the family.

A number of health visitors were worried that our visits to control mothers would raise their anxiety about cot death, especially since their baby would be the same age as the one who had died. We always gave control mothers the opportunity to ask questions and discuss their fears, and it was our impression that we raised their awareness but not their anxiety.

General practitioners had all been officially informed about the study, but they reported few deaths to us because most babies dying at home are taken directly to hospital by ambulance. Occasionally, a general practitioner would certify a death at home and the baby would be taken direct to a mortuary, which might cause delay in notification. Other problems sometimes encountered with general practitioners were opposition to our visiting early, and reluctance to provide copies of their notes for the confidential enquiry. However, in most cases general practitioners were very helpful, allowing access to their records and sharing their knowledge about the baby and family.

Local case discussion

After the parents had completed their part of the questionnaire, the researcher obtained additional information from any relevant medical notes, the only difficulty being when general practitioners refused access. When the full autopsy results were available, usually about eight weeks after the baby's death, the researcher helped to organise the local case discussion, which normally involved the general practitioner, health visitor, paediatrician and pathologist. Getting all these busy people together was a logistic nightmare, and the general practitioner's surgery at lunch time usually proved to be the most productive venue. For the researchers, the local case discussion served to round off our involvement with each family, completing the picture and assuring us that ongoing support was reliably in hand.

Personal impressions

Participation in the SUDI study was an exceptional experience, both professionally and personally. First visits to newly bereaved parents drew heavily upon our emotional resources, and although visits to control families helped to restore our perspective, we could not have survived without our network of mutual support. As the study progressed, it was gratifying to see the importance with which it was regarded and to join in the presentation of results. At the end, it was hard to go back to the routine of mainstream health visiting.

Summary of recommendations

- A background in health visiting is ideal for this type of research.
- Interviewers should all be in post prior to the piloting stage.
- Continuity is important and short-term temporary contracts are not suitable for projects of this kind.
- Time should be devoted to team-building at the start of the project.
- Interviewers should have regular clinical supervision and support, both individually and as a group.
- A flexible schedule is essential for this kind of work.

Chapter 7

CONCLUSIONS AND RECOMMENDATIONS

Peter Fleming, Peter Blair, Chris Bacon, Martin Ward Platt and Jem Berry

Introduction

The conclusions from the three main parts of the SUDI cases – case-control study, pathology investigations and confidential enquiry – have been summarised in the relevant chapters. From these conclusions recommendations can be made that are of importance to parents of small children and their families, to healthcare professionals, to health authorities and educators, to coroners and to the general public. The recommendations come under two main headings:

- prevention of sudden unexpected death in infancy;
- investigation and procedures following sudden unexpected death in infancy.

PREVENTION OF SUDDEN UNEXPECTED DEATH IN INFANCY

Training and targeting

The training of healthcare professionals who work with families and babies should include, at every stage, the latest information on factors that influence the risk of sudden death in infancy. Despite the success of the 'Back to Sleep' campaign, the SUDI study shows that not all healthcare professionals have incorporated key messages into their everyday practice.

In addition, it is apparent that information about risk factors is failing to reach or to be acted upon by that small minority of the population in which a disproportionate number of sudden infant deaths occur. Health education campaigns designed to reduce infant mortality must therefore be targeted, with appropriate evaluation, at the groups at greatest risk.

Potentially modifiable risk factors for SIDS

The results of the case-control study have provided better understanding of the risks and benefits of various aspects of infant care, confirming as risk factors for SIDS several items that had been previously suggested, whilst refuting (or failing to confirm) a number of others.

For other factors, the results of the study are inconclusive, and further research is needed before definite recommendations can be made.

Items that were confirmed or identified as risk factors

Sleeping position

The risk of SIDS is highest for infants sleeping in the prone position, and lowest for those in the supine position. The side position carries an intermediate risk, which is significantly higher than that of the supine position. Thus, infants should be placed to sleep on the back, not on the front or side. Extending the lower arm has little effect on the risk of sleeping in the side position.

Tobacco smoke

Infants should be protected from exposure to tobacco smoke during pregnancy and after birth. Parents should be encouraged to cut down or stop smoking during (or preferably before) pregnancy, and to create a smoke-free environment for the baby after birth.

The cot environment

Infants should not be heavily wrapped, should not lie on or be covered by duvets or quilts, and they should not wear hats indoors. Parents should be encouraged to adjust the bedding and clothing to maintain an environment in which the infant is neither too hot nor too cold. They should check by feeling the infant's chest or abdomen – this should feel warm but not sweaty. The bedding should be arranged so that it cannot ride up over the infant's head, and the infant should be placed in the 'feet to foot' position in the cot. Pillows, cushions and bean bags should not be used.

Room-sharing

Parents should be encouraged to share a bedroom with their baby for the first six months after birth.

Bed-sharing

Parents who smoke, have been drinking alcohol or using legal or illegal drugs (particularly those which may alter consciousness level or responsiveness), or are excessively tired should not share a bed with their baby for sleep.

Sofa-sharing

Parents should not share a sofa, settee or armchair with their baby to sleep at any time. Whilst sofas or armchairs are comfortable places to cuddle and feed infants, parents should be aware of the potential dangers of falling asleep there with the baby, particularly if they have recently consumed alcohol.

Illness recognition

Parents should be taught to recognise significant features of illness in babies, (e.g. by using the Cambridge 'Baby Check' system*), and to seek medical attention early if the baby is unwell.

Immunisation

Parents should be informed that immunisation does not increase the risk of SIDS, and that infants who are fully immunised are at a significantly lower risk of SIDS than those who are not immunised.

---

* Copies of the Baby Check scoring system can be obtained from: Baby Check, PO Box 324 Wroxham, Norwich NR12 8EQ. Tel: 01603 784400.

Items that were not confirmed as risk (or protective) factors, or that may have other adverse effects

Breast-feeding

Whilst the benefits to the infant from breast-feeding for as long a time as possible have been clearly shown in many studies, we could not find any evidence of an independent effect of breast-feeding in reducing the risk of SIDS. Breast-feeding should be strongly encouraged, but it is incorrect to use a reduction in the risk of SIDS as a reason to do so.

Dummies (pacifiers)

Whilst the data from this study confirm previous findings of an apparent reduction in the risk of SIDS for infants who use dummies, the adverse effects of dummies on the prevalence and duration of breast-feeding, and the increased incidence of respiratory and gastro-intestinal infections mean that further studies are needed before the use of a dummy can be advocated as a protective measure against SIDS.

Bed-sharing

Whilst there are certain circumstances in which bed-sharing with an adult is potentially hazardous for infants (see above), this study *did not* find any evidence of an increased risk of SIDS for infants who shared a bed with non-smoking parents.

Cot bumpers

Neither adverse effects nor benefits from the use of cot bumpers were identified in this study.

Apnoea monitors

Whilst such devices are widely used, both for the purpose of reassuring parents and their supposed benefits to the infant, we found no evidence that such devices are of any value in preventing SIDS.

Mattress type or age (the 'toxic gas' hypothesis)

As previously published in the Limerick Report, the CESDI study found no evidence to support this hypothesis. The risk of SIDS was *not* increased by the use of an older mattress, and was *lower* for infants who slept on mattresses with PVC covers. Antimony concentrations in hair were commonly found to be higher in infants than in their mothers, but this resulted from prenatal accumulation rather than from contamination by mattresses [1].

Aeroplane flights or trips to high altitude

This study found no evidence to support the hypothesis that long-haul air flights are a significant contributory factor to SIDS.

Recommendations: families at risk, babies at risk and circumstances of risk

A picture has emerged of certain features of the family, the baby and the circumstances which are associated with increased risk of SIDS. Some of these features are potentially more amenable to change, whilst other features may serve as 'markers' of the family, or infant, at risk and may be used by health care professionals to target appropriate health care and advice.

Factors for health care professionals to note

Factors which are likely to be amenable to change by advice from healthcare professionals:

Encourage

- supine sleeping position for infants;
- placing the infant in the cot in the 'feet to foot' position;
- sharing a room with the baby for the first six months.

Discourage

- sleeping with the infant on a sofa, settee or armchair;
- bed-sharing when parents are tired or have taken drugs to help them sleep;
- heavy wrapping and high room temperature;
- the use of pillows, duvets or loose bedding (particularly if there is a risk of inadvertent head covering).

Factors which may be amenable to modification by advice from healthcare professionals, but which involve a change in parental behaviour:

Encourage

- immunisation.

Discourage

- exposure of pregnant women and infants to cigarette smoke;
- bed-sharing by parents who have recently consumed alcohol or illicit drugs.

Factors which, whilst potentially amenable to change, will require the development of a strategy to achieve a significant change in parental behaviour include:

- maternal smoking during pregnancy;
- bed-sharing and smoking;
- parental alcohol or other drug abuse.

Factors which may alert healthcare professionals to the special needs of the family include:

- low maternal age;[*]
- high maternal parity (particularly if mother is under 25);[*]
- low income;[*]
- maternal smoking during pregnancy;[*]
- smoking in the home;
- poor or crowded housing;
- single unsupported mother;

---

[*] Three of these four factors are present in 8% of the population in general, but in over 40% of SIDS families.

- baby of low birth weight, short gestation or multiple birth;

- baby with congenital anomaly;

- recent move of house (especially during the year before the birth).

Whilst there is no direct evidence that improvement of social conditions decreases the risk of SIDS, the strong association of socio-economic deprivation and poor housing with SIDS should encourage health care professionals to work with colleagues in the social services to try to improve housing conditions for such families whenever possible.

Acute factors which may signify transient increased risk and alert family or healthcare professionals to the need for close observation or possible treatment include:

- a high 'Baby Check' score;

- a history of an apparent life-threatening event.

Factors for parents to note

While it is not possible to guarantee that any baby will not be a victim of cot death, the risk can be substantially reduced by following certain simple guidelines:

- Place your baby to sleep on his/her back, not the front or side.

- Place your baby on a clean dry mattress. Use lightweight blankets and clothing. Avoid the use of duvets, quilts, pillows, cushions or bean bags. Check your baby to ensure that he/she does not feel too hot or too cold.

- Place your baby to sleep so that his/her feet are close to the foot of the cot ('feet to foot') with the bedding securely tucked in and no higher than the baby's chin.

- Never sleep with your baby on a sofa, settee or armchair. If you cuddle or feed your baby on a sofa, settee or armchair, ensure you do not fall asleep with him/her.

- If possible, place your baby's cot in the same room as your bed.

- While it is safe to take your baby into bed with you to feed or for comfort, there are certain circumstances, especially in the first four months of life, when it is important to place him/her back in the cot before you go to sleep. These include:

  – if you or your partner smoke;

  – if you or your partner have recently consumed alcohol;

  – if you or your partner have recently taken drugs which make you sleep more heavily;

  – if you or your partner are extremely tired.

  Unlike cots, adult beds and bunk-beds are not designed to meet safety standards for infants. Bunk-beds pose particular risks of injury to young infants who can slip under the side safety bar and be strangled.

  If you plan to sleep with your baby, make sure the baby's head cannot become covered by bedding. Keep the baby away from the pillows, use lightweight blankets rather than adult bed covers (e.g. duvets) and place your baby in a position where there is no risk of him/her falling out of the bed.

- Do not smoke during pregnancy or go into a room in which others are smoking. If you cannot completely stop, then cut down as much as possible.

- Do not smoke in any room in which young infants ever go. Keep your baby out of rooms in which people smoke (in other words, maintain a 'smoke-free zone' around yourself whilst pregnant, and around your baby after he/she is born).

- If your baby is unwell, particularly if he/she has a temperature, has any difficulty breathing or is less responsive than usual, seek medical help promptly.

INVESTIGATION AND PROCEDURES FOLLOWING SUDDEN UNEXPECTED DEATHS IN INFANCY

Introduction

Recent authoritative commentaries from the United Kingdom [2–5] and from the United States [6] have argued that present arrangements for the investigation of sudden infant deaths are inadequate and in need of revision. Many of the findings in the SUDI study, which is the most comprehensive study of its kind yet undertaken in the UK, support these contentions. In particular, deficiencies have been demonstrated in current arrangements for the examination of the circumstances of the death and the collection of all relevant information (Chapter 5), and for the post-mortem examination and accurate certification (Chapter 4). As a result, the opportunities for determining the true cause of death, where this is possible, are not fully exploited, so that parents may not be properly advised, official statistics may be wrong, and vulnerable children may sometimes be left unprotected. In addition, families may not always be treated with the informed sensitivity that their bereavement requires (Chapter 6).

We propose below a revised system for investigation and procedures following sudden deaths in infancy that is based on the experience of the SUDI studies. Many of our recommendations have already been made in previous reports by the National Advisory Body for CESDI (Appendix I). So far as possible, our proposals conform to the present system, while seeking to remedy the shortcomings that have been demonstrated within it.

Proposed new arrangements

Collection of information

As soon as possible after the death, ideally within 24–48 hours, all relevant information should be collected from the parents or carers. This information should include detailed accounts of the events leading up to the death and the circumstances in which it occurred, the previous health of the child and other family members, and the family's social and economic background. The interview with the parents should be conducted by a senior health care professional, such as a paediatrician, a general practitioner, or a specially trained health visitor who has knowledge and experience of child care, disease in childhood and bereavement. Since the majority of sudden infant deaths do not result from unlawful actions, it is not appropriate that this initial collection of information is normally or solely carried out by a police officer. An experienced health care professional is trained to recognise any suggestion of maltreatment and to consult with other agencies, including the police, at an early stage.

The SUDI studies have shown that an early interview that is sympathetic and well informed not only yields the most accurate information but also helps the family to start coming to terms with what has happened to them. In addition to the interview with parents, information must also be collected from all other relevant sources, such as the general practitioner and health visitor, maternity and hospital records, and social services departments.

Each health trust or district should designate one or more people to carry out this role of interviewing and collecting information. In view of the reduced frequency of sudden infant deaths, it may be appropriate for interviewers to serve more than one district, and it will be helpful if all those designated within a region meet regularly for the purposes of training and mutual support.

A copy of the interviewer's report could routinely be sent to the coroner. With regard to the police, it would seem to be most appropriate if liaison over sudden infant deaths and any ensuing police inquiries were normally carried out by officers designated for child protection. These officers will be particularly experienced in dealing with families, in recognising maltreatment, and in working with health professionals.

Post-mortem examination

A large majority of unexpected deaths in infancy result from natural causes, which may occasionally include inherited disorders that have vital implications for the family. Parents who have suffered a cot death want to know above all why their baby died, and they have a right to expect that everything possible is done to answer their question. The data set out in Table 4.1 show that at present this does not always happen. We therefore strongly endorse previous recommendations [7–9] that all post-mortem examinations of infants who have died suddenly and unexpectedly should be carried out by a paediatric pathologist, or by a general pathologist with special training and expertise. When appropriate, the examination may be carried out jointly with a forensic pathologist, but it should not be conducted solely by a forensic pathologist unless he or she has had special training in paediatric pathology.

Before he or she begins the post-mortem examination, the pathologist should be fully briefed on the history and on the circumstances of the death by the person who has interviewed the parents and collected other data as described above. The SUDI pathologists concluded that such a briefing was the single most important factor in enabling them to make a correct diagnosis, but under present arrangements it is often badly deficient. Inadequate briefing may result in failure to carry out the tests that might lead to the identification of a cause of death, whether natural or unnatural. The examination should follow a recommended minimum protocol, with additions according to particular circumstances.

Now that the number of sudden infant deaths has decreased, it is more feasible to refer all cases for specialist autopsy. This is already done in some regions, delays being kept to a minimum by good communication and allocation of high priority.

Multidisciplinary case discussion

The SUDI study has confirmed the value of holding a multidisciplinary case discussion after every unexpected death in infancy. The meeting should normally take place in the primary care setting a few weeks after the death, and should be attended by all the relevant professionals, including the general practitioner, the health visitor, the designated interviewer, a paediatrician (who may also be the interviewer), the pathologist, plus, when appropriate, other professionals such as midwife and social worker.

The meeting would have several purposes: to examine all the details of the death, including the final results of post-mortem investigations, and to agree on the most likely cause and contributory factors; if there was any suggestion of maltreatment, to apply the appropriate procedures for child protection, including consultation with the social services department and with the police; to see whether there had been errors or deficiencies in professional care and surveillance, and whether lessons could be learned for the future; to see whether the carers would benefit from additional guidance and support in their child care practices; and to ensure that the needs of all the family for help in their bereavement were being adequately met, and that they would be fully advised and supported in any future pregnancy. Although the parents would not attend this meeting themselves, it is important that one of the professionals concerned should meet them soon afterwards to discuss the conclusions and implications (ideally a written summary, in appropriate terms, should also be given), and to answer questions. A formal report could also be provided for the coroner.

Certification of the cause of death

When a baby has died unexpectedly, the family needs to know the cause as soon as possible, both for emotional and for practical reasons. However, the cause may sometimes not become apparent, or classification as SIDS cannot properly be made, until the results of all pathological and other investigations are known, which will usually take about six weeks. This dilemma might best be resolved if, in those cases (which will be the majority) where the cause of death is not immediately apparent from the circumstances or from the autopsy, the death certificate initially issued is designated as provisional. A final certificate can then be issued after all investigations have been completed and the multidisciplinary discussion has been held. For deaths in which the cause is immediately apparent, there need be no provisional certificate and a final certificate can be issued at once.

If provisional certification were adopted as standard practice in all cases that were initially uncertain, and if parents were appropriately informed and advised, the distress and stigmatisation that may now accompany delay in certification could be largely avoided. The parents would need to be sensitively supported through this difficult interim period, preferably by one of the professionals participating in the case discussion.

As at present, these procedures would be under the control of the coroner.

Advantages of these proposals

The measures proposed above would bring the following benefits:

- They would make it more likely that the cause of natural death is found in those cases where this is possible.
- They would make it more likely that deaths resulting from maltreatment are identified.
- They would lead to more accurate certification of death in infancy, and so to greater accuracy in official statistics.
- They would ensure that bereaved parents are given all appropriate support and information as early as possible.
- They would enable lessons to be learned about the care given by professionals or by parents that might improve the welfare of future infants.

Implementation

The practicality of most of these proposals has already been demonstrated by their successful operation in various parts of the UK, both during and outside the SUDI studies. However, investigation and procedures following sudden infant deaths vary widely in different areas, often being determined by the views of influential individuals. A move towards a standard national approach will require agreement about respective areas of responsibility and about funding between coroners, police, health authorities, paediatricians and pathologists. Although the measures proposed could be largely incorporated within the present system, there will be a need for firm central guidance, possibly backed by legislation.

Little extra funding would be required because, apart from the specialist interviewers, the measures would make use of existing resources. A pilot study conducted in 1998 in Avon, which has a population of approximately one million, suggests that interviewing and data collection might require, for example, one session a week from a designated health visitor with support from a consultant paediatrician. We consider that this is a small outlay for the important benefits to be gained from the proposed new system.

Conclusion

This report strongly recommends that the Home Office and the Department of Health should review the present system of investigation and other procedures following sudden deaths in infancy and should consider the early introduction of the measures outlined above.

References

1. Fleming, PJ, Blair, P, Cooke, M, Warnock, D, Berry, PJ, Smith, I, Thompson, M, Ward-Platt, M and Hall, D. 'Studies to establish whether antimony or other chemicals added to cot mattress covers are of significance in the aetiology of sudden infant death' in *The Report of the Expert Group to Investigate Cot Death Theories: Toxic Gas Hypothesis*. London: Department of Health, 1998.

2. Meadow, R. 'Unnatural sudden infant death', *Archives of Diseases in Childhood*, 1999; 80: 7–14.

3. Editorial (anon). 'Unexplained deaths in infancy', *Lancet*, 1999; 353: 161.

4. Green, MA. 'Time to put "cot death" to bed?', *British Medical Journal*, 1999; 319: 697–8.

5. Limerick, S. 'Not time to put cot death to bed', *British Medical Journal*, 1999; 319: 698–700.

6. Centers for Disease Control and Prevention. *Guidelines for Death Scene Investigation of Sudden, Unexplained Infant Deaths: Recommendations of the Interagency Panel on Sudden Infant Death Syndrome*. Atlanta, USA: Morbidity and Mortality Weekly Report, 1996; 45 (no. RR-10): 1–22.

7. Brodrick committee. *Report of the Committee on Death Certification and Coroners*. London HMSO, 1971: Cmnd 4810; Brodrick report.

8. Knowelden, J, Keeling, J and Nicholl, JP. A *Multicentre Study of Post-neonatal Mortality*. University of Sheffield: Medical Care Research Unit, 1985.

9. Clothier, Sir Cecil. *The Allitt Inquiry: Independent Inquiry Relating to Deaths and Injuries on the Children's Ward at Grantham and Kesteven General Hospital During the Period February to April 1991*. London: HMSO, 1994.

APPENDIX I

PAST RECOMMENDATIONS FROM CESDI ABOUT RELEVANT PROFESSIONAL AND SERVICE ISSUES

Various recommendations about professional and service issues were made in the Third and Fifth Annual Reports for CESDI [1,2]. These are summarised below. The bracketed numbers refer to sections from the CESDI reports; the first number denotes whether the reference is to the Third or the Fifth Report.

Recommendations that concern all health professionals

1. All relevant health professionals should keep themselves informed about current knowledge of the factors that affect the risk of cot death, and should routinely advise mothers and other carers accordingly. (3. 9.3.1)

2. Advice should be given in such a way that recipients are most likely to accept and respond to it. (3. 9.3.2)

3. Any professional who has concerns about the welfare of a child should consult with other properly interested parties, with due regard for confidentiality. (3. 9.3.8)

4. All professionals should keep clear and adequate notes. (3. 9.3.10)

5. Any health professional who may have responsibility for the care of sick babies should be trained in the emergency cardio-pulmonary resuscitation of infants. (5. 4.4.1)

Recommendations about general practice

1. All general practitioners should receive training in the recognition of serious illness in babies. (3. 9.3.3 and 5. 4.4.1)

2. General practitioners should be encouraged to play their full part in properly authorised confidential enquiries, including provision of their records. (3. 9.3.11)

Recommendations about paediatric departments

1. Continuing education for consultant paediatricians should include the best current management of acute severe illness in infancy. (5. 4.4.1)

2. A consultant community paediatrician (or other appropriate professional) should be designated in each district or trust to take the lead role in coordinating supervision and support for families whose children are thought to be vulnerable, for monitoring sudden infant deaths and in coordinating the response to them. (3. 9.3.8 and 9.6.7)

3. Paediatric departments should ensure that any sick baby brought to hospital, including to a casualty department, is always assessed by a sufficiently experienced doctor before being sent home. (5. 4.4.2)

4. Paediatric departments should liaise with midwifery departments to ensure that all babies, including those born at home, receive a proper medical examination in the first week of life. (3. 9.2.12)

Recommendations about health visiting

Health visitors should target their service, giving extra supervision and support to vulnerable and disadvantaged families. (5. 4.4.2)

Recommendations about the response to sudden infant death

1. A network should be established in each district or trust to ensure that all sudden infant deaths are notified to the designated paediatrician as soon as possible. (3. 9.6.7)

2. Prior to the autopsy, the pathologist should be fully briefed. In compiling his report, the coroner's officer should consult with the designated paediatrician, or failing this should follow a checklist of points that need to be covered. (3. 9.5.1)

3. Whenever possible, autopsies on babies who have died suddenly and unexpectedly should be carried out by a specialist paediatric pathologist, in cooperation with a forensic pathologist when this is considered necessary. If a specialist is not available, the pathologist should follow the recommended protocol for infant autopsies. (3. 9.4.3–5 and 10)

4. Following any sudden unexpected death in infancy, the designated paediatrician should convene a local case discussion to discuss all aspects of the death, especially the provision of continuing support to the family, possible causes of death and lessons for the future. Participants should include the general practitioner, health visitor, pathologist and paediatrician. (3. 9.6.8)

References

1. Department of Health. *Confidential Enquiry into Stillbirths and Deaths in Infancy: Third Annual Report*. London: DoH, 1996.

2. Department of Health. *Confidential Enquiry into Stillbirths and Deaths in Infancy: Fifth Annual Report*. London: Maternal and Child Health Consortium, 1998.

APPENDIX II

PREVIOUS PUBLICATIONS FROM THE CESDI SUDI STUDIES

1. Blair, P, Fleming, PJ, Bensley, D, Smith, I, Bacon, C and Taylor, E. 'Plastic mattresses and sudden infant death syndrome', *Lancet*, 1995; 345: 720.

2. Blair, P, Fleming, PJ, Bensley, D, Smith, I, Bacon, C, Taylor, E, Berry, PJ and Tripp, J. 'The SUDI Case-Control Study' in *The Annual Report for 1994 of the National Advisory Body for CESDI*. London: Department of Health, 1996.

3. Fleming, PJ, Blair, P, Bacon, C, Bensley, D, Smith, I, Taylor, E, Berry, PJ, Golding, J and Tripp, J. 'The environment of infants during sleep and the risk of sudden infant death syndrome: results of 1993–5 case-control study for confidential enquiry into stillbirths and deaths in infancy', *British Medical Journal*, 1996; 313: 191–5.

4. Blair, P, Fleming, PJ, Bensley, D, Smith, I, Bacon, C, Taylor, E, Berry, PJ, Golding, J and Tripp, J. 'Smoking and sudden infant death syndrome: results of 1993–5 case-control study for confidential enquiry into stillbirths and deaths in infancy', *British Medical Journal*, 1996; 313: 195–8.

5. Fleming, PJ, Blair, P, Cooke, M, Warnock, D, Berry, PJ, Smith, I, Thompson, M, Ward-Platt, M and Hall, D. 'Studies to establish whether antimony or other chemicals added to cot mattress covers are of significance in the aetiology of sudden infant death' in *The Report of the Expert Group to Investigate Cot Death Theories: Toxic Gas Hypothesis*. London: Department of Health, 1998: Appendix III.

6. Ward-Platt, MP, Blair, PS, Leach, CEA, Smith, I and Fleming, PJ. 'Danger to babies from air travel must be small', *British Medical Journal*, 1998; 317: 676–7.

7. Bacon C, Blair, P, Leach, CEA, Fleming, PJ, Smith, I, Ward-Platt, M and Hall, D. 'Sudden Infant Deaths other than SIDS' in *Report on CESDI*. London: The Maternal and Child Health Research Consortium, 1998.

8. Leach, CEA, Blair, PS, Fleming, PJ, Smith, IJ, Ward-Platt, M, Berry, PJ and Golding, J. 'Sudden Unexpected Deaths in Infancy: Similarities and Differences in the Epidemiology of SIDS and Explained Deaths', *Pediatrics Electronic Pages*, 1999; 104: e43.

9. Fleming, PJ, Blair, PS, Pollard, K, Platt, MW, Leach, C, Smith, I, Berry, PJ and Golding, J. 'Pacifier use and SIDS – results from the CESDI SUDI case-control study', *Archives of Diseases in Childhood*, 1999; 81(2): 112–16.

10. Ward-Platt, M, Blair, PS, Fleming, PJ, Smith, IJ, Cole, TJ, Leach, CEA and Golding, J. 'Sudden Unexpected Death in Infancy: a clinical comparison of explained and unexplained deaths – how healthy and how normal?', *Archives of Diseases in Childhood*, 1999 (in press).

11. Blair, PS, Fleming, PJ, Smith, IJ, Platt, MW, Young, J, Nadin, P, Berry, PJ and Golding, J, the CESDI SUDI research group and Mitchell, E. 'Babies sleeping with parents: case-control factors influencing the risk of sudden infant death syndrome', *British Medical Journal*, 1999; 319: 1457–62.

12. Blair, PS, Nadin, P, Cole, TJ, Fleming, PJ, Smith, IJ, Ward-Platt, M, Berry, PJ and Golding, J. 'Weight gain and Sudden Infant Death Syndrome', *Archives of Diseases in Childhood*, 1999 (in press).

INDEX

Page numbers in italic indicate reference to a figure

UNIVERSITY OF WOLVERHAMPTON LEARNING RESOURCES